T0252341

Person-centred Care in Radiography

Skills for Providing Effective Patient Care

First Edition

Ruth M. Strudwick DProf, MSc, BSc(Hons), CTCert, PGCE, SFHEA, FCR

Jane M. Harvey-Lloyd PhD, MSc, DCR(R) PGCE, DLC, CTC, RPS

Jill Bleiker PhD, MSc, BSc, PgCert, FHEA

Jane Gooch PGDip, PGCAPHE, BSc, BMus, FHEA

Amy Hancock PhD, MSc, BSc (Hons), PGCe, FHEA

Emma Hyde PhD, MEd, BSc (Hons), NTF, FHEA

Ann Newton-Hughes DProf, MSc, PGCT&L, DMU, DCR(R)

WILEY Blackwell

This edition first published 2024
© 2024 John Wiley & Sons Ltd

All rights reserved. No part of this publication may be reproduced, stored in a retrieval system, or transmitted, in any form or by any means, electronic, mechanical, photocopying, recording or otherwise, except as permitted by law. Advice on how to obtain permission to reuse material from this title is available at http://www.wiley.com/go/permissions.

The right of Ruth M. Strudwick, Jane M. Harvey-Lloyd, Jill Bleiker, Jane Gooch, Amy Hancock, Emma Hyde, and Ann Newton-Hughes to be identified as the authors of this work has been asserted in accordance with law.

Registered Office
John Wiley & Sons Ltd, The Atrium, Southern Gate, Chichester, West Sussex, PO19 8SQ, UK

For details of our global editorial offices, customer services, and more information about Wiley products visit us at www.wiley.com.

Wiley also publishes its books in a variety of electronic formats and by print-on-demand. Some content that appears in standard print versions of this book may not be available in other formats.

Trademarks: Wiley and the Wiley logo are trademarks or registered trademarks of John Wiley & Sons, Inc. and/or its affiliates in the United States and other countries and may not be used without written permission. All other trademarks are the property of their respective owners. John Wiley & Sons, Inc. is not associated with any product or vendor mentioned in this book.

Limit of Liability/Disclaimer of Warranty
The contents of this work are intended to further general scientific research, understanding, and discussion only and are not intended and should not be relied upon as recommending or promoting scientific method, diagnosis, or treatment by physicians for any particular patient. In view of ongoing research, equipment modifications, changes in governmental regulations, and the constant flow of information relating to the use of medicines, equipment, and devices, the reader is urged to review and evaluate the information provided in the package insert or instructions for each medicine, equipment, or device for, among other things, any changes in the instructions or indication of usage and for added warnings and precautions. While the publisher and authors have used their best efforts in preparing this work, they make no representations or warranties with respect to the accuracy or completeness of the contents of this work and specifically disclaim all warranties, including without limitation any implied warranties of merchantability or fitness for a particular purpose. No warranty may be created or extended by sales representatives, written sales materials or promotional statements for this work. This work is sold with the understanding that the publisher is not engaged in rendering professional services. The advice and strategies contained herein may not be suitable for your situation. You should consult with a specialist where appropriate. The fact that an organization, website, or product is referred to in this work as a citation and/or potential source of further information does not mean that the publisher and authors endorse the information or services the organization, website, or product may provide or recommendations it may make. Further, readers should be aware that websites listed in this work may have changed or disappeared between when this work was written and when it is read. Neither the publisher nor authors shall be liable for any loss of profit or any other commercial damages, including but not limited to special, incidental, consequential, or other damages.

Library of Congress Cataloging-in-Publication Data applied for

Paperback ISBN: 9781119833574

Cover image: © Isaac Lane Koval/Corbis/VCG/Getty Images; FS Productions/Getty Images; ER Productions Limited/Getty Images
Cover design by Wiley

Set in 10.5/13pt STIXTwoText by Straive, Chennai, India
Printed and bound by CPI Group (UK) Ltd, Croydon, CR0 4YY

C9781119833574_170823

Contents

List of Contributors

Ruth M. Strudwick DProf, MSc, BSc(Hons), CTCert, PGCE, SFHEA, FCR
Professor in Diagnostic Radiography
Head of AHP
School of Health and Sports Sciences
University of Suffolk
Ipswich, UK

Jane M. Harvey-Lloyd PhD, MSc, DCR(R), PGCE, DLC, CTC, RPS
Associate Professor
School of Health and Sports Sciences
University of Suffolk
Ipswich, UK

Jill Bleiker PhD, MSc, BSc, PgCert, FHEA
Honorary Senior Lecturer
Medical Imaging, University of Exeter Medical School
Exeter, UK

Jane Gooch PGDip, PGCAPHE, BSc, BMus, FHEA
Senior Lecturer
School of Allied Health and Social Care, College of Health, Psychology, and Social Care
University of Derby
Derby, UK

Amy Hancock PhD, MSc, BSc (Hons), PGCe, FHEA
Senior Lecturer
Medical Imaging, University of Exeter
Exeter, UK

Emma Hyde PhD, MEd, BSc (Hons), NTF, FHEA
Associate Professor
Provost for Learning and Teaching
University of Derby
Derby, UK

Ann Newton-Hughes DProf MSc PGCT&L DMU DCR(R)
Retired Lecturer
School of Health and Society
University of Salford
Salford, UK

CHAPTER 1

Introduction

Ruth M. Strudwick and Emma Hyde

Patient care is an important and sometimes overlooked part of the otherwise technical and mechanistic roles of the diagnostic and therapeutic radiographer. Increasing emphasis has been placed on the quality of care provided by all health professionals in publications such as the National Health Service (NHS) Five Year Forward View (NHS England 2014), The Long-term Plan (NHS England 2019) and the Health Foundation's Person-centred Care Made Simple document (The Health Foundation 2014) and this is driving changes in attitudes towards patient care. The Francis Report (Francis 2013) and 'Hello My Name is' campaign (Granger 2013), have also highlighted the need for improved communication skills to display compassion in health care. In radiography, the highly technical nature of the professional role can lead to a tension between image production or treatment delivery, and the time and personal resources available for patient care. The Covid-19 pandemic has heightened the emphasis on patient care skills and brought into sharp focus how the quality of the interaction between radiographer and patient can make a difference to the individual service user's experience.

There are several terms in common use when discussing the quality of care delivered by health and social care professionals. These terms are patient, person, or family-centred care. Patient- and family-centred care overlap significantly, and can be defined as:

"Patient and family centred care encourages the active collaboration and shared decision making between patients, families and providers to design and manage a customized and comprehensive care plan"

—NEJM Catalyst 2021

Person-centred Care in Radiography: Skills for Providing Effective Patient Care, First Edition.
Ruth M. Strudwick, Jane M. Harvey-Lloyd, Jill Bleiker, Jane Gooch, Amy Hancock, Emma Hyde, and Ann Newton-Hughes.
© 2024 John Wiley & Sons Ltd. Published 2024 by John Wiley & Sons Ltd.

Person-centred care has been evolving since the 1980s, starting with the work of the Picker Institute (Picker Institute Europe 2022), who strived to achieve their vision of:

"The highest quality person centred care for all, always."

The Health Foundation (2014) built upon this work to develop their definition of person-centred care:

"Person-centred care supports people to develop the knowledge, skills and confidence they need to more effectively manage and make informed decisions about their own health and health care."

Tensions between providing person-centred care and the UK NHS model of health and care delivery are particularly evident with imaging and radiotherapy services (Bleiker 2020). Reductionist approaches to patients and continued focus on the symptomatic body part or pathology being treated can result in a lack of holistic person-centred care. Advances in imaging and radiotherapy technologies are changing how services are delivered, enabling significant efficiency improvements, but this may be at the expense of person-centred care approaches. Examples are provided in Hyde & Hardy (2021) and Taylor (2020) of how radiography services can be perceived by service users which demonstrate the importance of person-centred approaches:

"I think, probably for radiographers more than quite a few other professions, they've got to be experts in something that's a bit more technical. They've got to be good at the technical, but maybe the communication thing is as much their skill set. It really needs to be worked on because from the patient's point of view they're both equally important."

—Diagnostic radiography patient

"They actually want to find out, find out how they can best help you and by finding out that and then doing that, that is the compassion side of it, as opposed to just a carte blanche or I'm really sorry or, you know, it is a way of going beyond that and saying, right, I want to find out how I can best help out that person."

—Therapeutic radiography patient

"You want the person [radiographer] to smile, to engage with you as a person, not purely [as] a patient. So sometimes it's just a few words, could be about the sort of time you took to get there or the weather or anything, it doesn't have to be formal, that's the main thing."

—Diagnostic radiography patient

"Be considerate really, they're a person, don't just view them as a body, going through this machine."

—Diagnostic radiographer

"And I think asking them how they feel as well because what might be important to one person isn't to another and its very individual to that patient."

—Therapeutic radiographer

Radiography professionals should ensure that as services change and adapt, person-centred approaches, and informed decision making, remain at the core of their day-to-day practice. Throughout this book we will use the term 'person-centred care' to encourage a more holistic view of the individuals we are providing imaging or radiotherapy services for. We may also use the terms 'patient' and 'service user', and this will depend on the context of the discussion. Not everyone accessing imaging or radiotherapy services is a patient, for example pregnant women attending for ultrasound imaging, or people attending a screening programme including the abdominal aortic aneurysm screening programme or the national breast screening programme.

This book will explore the complex interpersonal skills required of radiotherapy practitioners and medical imaging professionals that enable the provision of high-quality person-centred care in radiography. The book brings together the research, experiences, expertise, and interests of all the authors, and is targeted at all staff working within diagnostic and therapeutic radiography, whether in clinical departments or educational institutions. This includes radiographers, assistant practitioners, support workers, and administrative staff. This book can also be used in radiography education and training by both students and educators, and by clinical staff who wish to reflect on their own practice and develop their person-centred care skills.

This book is unique in that it is grounded in research undertaken by the authors. The authors' research explores service users', radiography students', and professionals' experiences to provide an evidence-based perspective on current practice, which combined with their clinical expertise, has been used to develop a book which promotes self-reflection, provides personal and professional development tools, and will help clinicians prepare to meet patients' expectations in clinical practice.

Throughout the book there are activities for readers to undertake to encourage self-discovery and reflection; the reader can then apply their learning to their own role. There are also scenarios developed by service users based on real-life practice, to demonstrate the impact of the professional's behaviour on the care received which allow reflection on person-centred approaches/values-based approaches. Diagrams and illustrations are used throughout the book to provide visual representation of the concepts presented.

REFERENCES

Bleiker, J. (2020). What radiographers talk about when they talk about compassion. *Journal of Medical Imaging and Radiation Sciences* 51 (4S): S44–S52. https://doi.org/10.1016/j.jmir.2020.08.009.

Francis, R. (2013). *Report of the Mid Staffordshire NHS Foundation Trust Public Inquiry*. London: The Stationery Office. https://www.gov.uk/government/publications/report-of-the-mid-staffordshire-nhs-foundation-trust-public-inquiry/ (accessed 22 February 2021).

Granger, K. (2013). Hello my name is campaign. https://www.hellomynameis.org.uk/ (accessed 22 January 2021).

Hyde, E. and Hardy, M. (2021). Delivering patient centred care (Part 2): a qualitative study of the perceptions of service users and deliverers. *Radiography* 27 (2): 322–331. https://doi.org/10.1016/j.radi.2020.09.008.

NEJM Catalyst (2021). What is patient-centred care? https://d.docs.live.net/f22ddaf61e56a367/Documents/Strudwick/To%20Copyeditor/Mechanical%20editing/c01/(nejm.org) (accessed 15 July 2021).

NHS England (2014). Five year forward view. https://www.england.nhs.uk/five-year-forward-view/ (accessed 29 October 2020).

NHS England (2019). The NHS long term plan. https://www.longtermplan.nhs.uk/publication/nhs-long-term-plan/ (accessed 29 October 2020).

Picker Institute Europe (2022). Principles of person centred care. https://www.picker.org/about-us/picker-principles-of-person-centred-care/ (accessed 11 October 2019).

Taylor, A. (2020). Defining compassion and compassionate behaviours in radio-therapy. Unpublished doctoral thesis. Sheffield Hallam University.

The Health Foundation (2014). Person-centred care made simple. `http://www.health.org.uk/sites/health/files/PersonCentredCareMadeSimple.pdf` (accessed 29 October 2020).

SECTION I

UNDERSTANDING OURSELVES

CHAPTER 2

Exploration of Your Own Values

Ruth M. Strudwick, Ann Newton-Hughes, and
Jane M. Harvey-Lloyd

Values and beliefs are intrinsically linked and form a part of who we are as a person. Beliefs are things that we hold as true and are usually formed in our childhood and are reinforced by our family, friends, and experiences throughout life. Often, they are not necessarily factually correct or can be proven (even if we believe them to be true) but they do influence who we are, what motivates us, and how we behave. They can often cause emotional turmoil within, and this can drive individuals to fight for what they believe.

Values are closely linked to our beliefs and often support these beliefs. We are usually less aware of our values than our beliefs, however they are just as important and help us to form our identity. They can be expressed in the form of our needs, wishes, preferences, and the things that are important to us. Our values are our principles or standards of behaviour; our judgement of what is important in life. Understanding our own values allows us to increase not only our self-awareness but to be more sensitive to recognising the values of others and how this influences their behaviour and the decisions that they may make. Having an awareness of values and in particular core values enable us to care more effectively for people as practitioners.

The Iceberg Model (Iceberg Principle 2011) (Figure 2.1) illustrates how values and beliefs directly influence our behaviour. It is important to

Person-centred Care in Radiography: Skills for Providing Effective Patient Care, First Edition.
Ruth M. Strudwick, Jane M. Harvey-Lloyd, Jill Bleiker, Jane Gooch, Amy Hancock,
Emma Hyde, and Ann Newton-Hughes.
© 2024 John Wiley & Sons Ltd. Published 2024 by John Wiley & Sons Ltd.

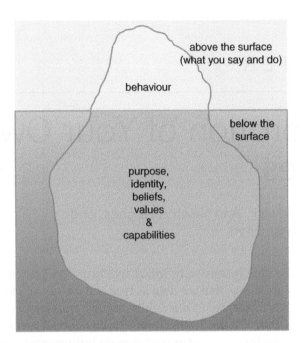

FIGURE 2.1   Iceberg model (Iceberg Principle 2011).

recognise that behaviour is only the tip of the iceberg, but as a person it is the very thing we are continuously judged on. Under the tip of the iceberg are values, beliefs, purpose, capabilities, and identity. This represents the internal dialogue, thoughts, and feelings, that each individual has that guide and controls our behaviour. Unfortunately, we are often too quick to judge others on their behaviour without fully understanding what lies beneath the tip of the iceberg. Being able to appreciate this and the effect that beliefs and values may have on your own behaviour will only enhance the way in which you practise and care for others.

WHY ARE VALUES IMPORTANT?

Values are important as they influence our thought processes and our priorities. Our values are unique and individual to us, and they may change in different circumstances. We see this in healthcare when patients are faced with life-changing events, and decisions need to be made about treatment options.

WHAT ARE YOUR VALUES – FORCED CHOICE EXERCISE

You choose:

- Imagine you have developed early symptoms of a potentially fatal disease ...
- The National Institute of Health and Care Excellence (NICE) has approved two possible treatments.
- TREATMENT A – gives you a guaranteed period of remission but no cure.
- TREATMENT B – gives you a 50:50 chance of 'kill or cure'.
- Your decision – **how long a period of remission** would you want from Treatment A to choose that treatment rather than go for the 50:50 'kill or cure' from Treatment B?

It is **your** decision ...

"How long a period of remission would **I** want from Treatment A to choose that treatment rather than go for the 50:50 "kill or cure" from Treatment B?'

- Write down **your own** answer, thinking about **your** decision from your own point of view and in your own particular circumstances.

The way that people answer this question can be surprisingly different. It might be assumed that younger people would choose a longer time span and older people would choose a shorter time span. The choice of the length of time is very dependent upon the individuals' values. Some younger people chose one year with a rationale that they would live their life to the full during that time, others chose 70 years as they wish to see what the future holds for them.

Examples

Choice: 15 years
Rationale: I have two children and I want to know if they meet their career and personal aspirations. 15 years should be enough to know this.
This reflects one of my core values which is my family.

Choice: Three years

Rationale: I have always wanted to travel and see some of the world. Three years would allow me to finish my degree and travel with my friends.

This reflects my core values of friends and new experiences.

Identifying and reflecting on your core values, allows you to understand who you are as a person and what life means to you. People who are aware of their values and honour them in the way in which they live on a regular basis will lead a more fulfilling life. There will be many times as a practitioner that you will have your values challenged and will be asked to do something which does not align with your values. This can frequently make you feel uncomfortable and at times you might be unsure about how to react. The important thing to acknowledge about values is that they are not morals, there is no sense of right/wrong or of positive/negative. They are also intrinsic to the individual and not consciously chosen. They do, however, underpin everything that we do and play a significant role in our life.

Each person has a hierarchy of values which are reinforced by a range of beliefs. Fundamentally, this affects our decision-making and the way in which we behave.

There is a range of exercises that you can undertake to establish your values. Start with undertaking the exercise below:

Establishing values exercise:

Identify three people who have had the greatest impact on your life. What specific advice or value has remained with you?

Name:	Value:
Name:	Value:
Name:	Value:

List three books, films, poems, sayings, or music tracks that have contributed to your values. What insight has stuck with you?

Resource:	Insight:
Resource:	Insight:
Resource:	Insight:

List five peak experiences that have profoundly shaped your life/ career direction:

Experience	Value:
Experience	Value:
Experience	Value:
Experience	Value:
Experience	Value:

Now, you have begun to start thinking about your values, it is important to identify your core values – those that matter to you the most. This will help you to understand what drives and motivates you and allow you to consider that from another person's perspective. Complete the following exercise:

Core values exercise:

For each value you identify, consider what that value gives you, what does it mean to you? It is also important to establish where the value came from and how long you have had that value.

Finally, evaluate each of your values in terms of how important it is, then rank each value in order of personal significance.

Is there anything that has surprised you at all about undertaking this exercise and what do you think you can take forward from this?

If you have found it difficult to identify your values, there is a list at the end of the chapter which you may find useful as a prompt.

Values-based Practice (VBP) is the consideration of the individual patient's values in making decisions about their care. By patient's values we mean the unique preferences, concerns, and expectations each patient brings to a practice encounter which must be integrated into any decisions about the care of the patient. VBP takes into account and highlights what matters, and therefore is important to the patient (Fulford et al. 2012). As practitioners, we should not be making assumptions about what the patient wants, or indeed, reflect our own values upon the patients we image or treat as radiographers.

We can do this in practice by asking the patient to tell us what is important to them and providing them with enough information so that they can make informed choices. This is a critical aspect of true person-centred care and VBP.

Values can, and do vary, sometimes widely between individuals and between patient and practitioner. They are not fixed and may change over time and as life experiences accumulate. The crucial thing to remember is that as a practitioner you should not make assumptions about your patient's values, instead take the time if needed to ascertain what matters to them at that moment in time with regard to the task in hand, be that acquisition of a diagnostic image or delivery of a treatment fraction.

Other people's values need to be respected. In Chapter 5 of this book, we discuss the impact of pain on a patient and how this affects their judgement, and we also discuss values-based practice in more detail in Chapter 12 of the book.

We have recognised that our behaviours are based on beliefs and as such the values we display in our personal lives may not match with those required in our professional role. Therefore, we may have to manage our values to behave in a professional manner and to avoid judging others as a result of their differing values. Likewise, patients may feel that they need to manage or surrender their values in order to receive appropriate care. Our professional status and knowledge automatically place us in a position of power in relation to our patients who do not hold the same understanding of our procedures and practice (Corless et al. 2016). As radiographers we control who enters our areas of practice and patients are only allowed to enter once given permission. Even our presentation of standing when they are seated can add to this perceived mismatch in power. We need to ensure that this perceived imbalance of power does not prevent patients from expressing their values. This can be achieved by being welcoming and friendly, inviting the patient to express their values and by listening and acting accordingly.

As can be seen, from the information presented above, each person has their own values built on beliefs, experience, and capability. As a radiographer it is essential that we recognise our own values and that of our patients so that we can provide care which recognises each individual and their needs. We should strive to address any imbalance in our professional relationship with our patients to ensure that their needs are met while they are in our care.

LIST OF POTENTIAL VALUES

Acceptance	Fairness	Optimism
Accuracy	Flexibility	Patience
Acknowledgement	Focus	Personal growth
Authenticity	Freedom	Power
Beauty	Health	Quality
Belonging	Honesty	Reliability
Challenge	Humour	Religion
Choice	Independence	Respect
Communication	Integrity	Responsibility
Community	Joy	Risk Taking
Compassion	Justice	Romance
Creativity	Kindness	Spirituality
Empathy	Leadership	Success
Empowerment	Learning	Trust
Equality	Love	Truth
Excellence	Nurturing	

REFERENCES

Corless, L., Buckley, A., and Mee, S. (2016). Patient narratives 3: power inequalities between patients and nurses. *Nursing Times* 112: 12, 20–21.

Fulford, K.W.M., Peile, E., and Carroll, H. (2012). *Essentials of Values-based Practice: Clinical Stories Linking Science with people*. Cambridge: Cambridge University Press.

Iceberg Principle (2011). https://steps2sustainability.wordpress.com/tag/iceberg-model/ (accessed 14 April 2023).

Zeus, P. and Skiffington, S. (2000). *The Complete Guide to Coaching at Work*. North Ryde, NSW, Australia: McGraw-Hill Australia.

CHAPTER 3

Developing Resilience

Jane M. Harvey-Lloyd

THE NEED FOR RESILIENCE

Resilience is a now much discussed phenomenon amongst healthcare professionals, with both employers and employees beginning to acknowledge its importance and the need to develop this within the workplace. The pressures and stressors of working in today's National Health Service (NHS) do not discriminate and therefore students, newly qualified radiographers, and even the most experienced healthcare practitioners all need the ability to adopt personal and professional resilience.

The role of the radiographer is ever changing in response to advancing technology and the rising demand for imaging and cancer services (NHS Confederation 2014; Borras et al. 2016). An ageing population has led to an increase in patients with long term conditions with complex comorbidities, demanding different approaches from health professionals whilst stretching the NHS to its limit. The impact of increasing targets also adds to the daily pressure that health service providers face whilst they endeavour to adopt more effective and efficient ways of working. Resilience is not only something which current practitioners can find helpful to adopt for their own health and well-being, but it is also necessary to ensure effective and patient-centred services which can respond quickly to change.

McAllister and McKinnon (2009) highlight the pressures placed upon health professionals such as fast-paced work, interactions with a diverse range of people at different levels, the constant change, and the underpinning

Person-centred Care in Radiography: Skills for Providing Effective Patient Care, First Edition.
Ruth M. Strudwick, Jane M. Harvey-Lloyd, Jill Bleiker, Jane Gooch, Amy Hancock,
Emma Hyde, and Ann Newton-Hughes.
© 2024 John Wiley & Sons Ltd. Published 2024 by John Wiley & Sons Ltd.

desire to care for others. It is this 'desire to care' that makes health and social care professions stand out from any other type of career in that most people tend to enter these professions *'because they sincerely want to care for others'* (Skovolt 2001). In doing so, the emotional energy/labour that this requires may lead to stress-related issues and evidence suggests that health professions suffer more from this type of issue in the workplace in comparison with other professions (Mann 2005; Wieclaw et al. 2006).

ACTIVITY 3.1

Make a list of all the challenges you will face as a student/qualified radiographer which challenge your resilience.

When you have made your list, grade the severity of the challenge from 0–10, with 0 being no challenge and 10 being a very strong challenge. Identify your top three challenges and think about what you can do to minimise the impact these may have on your resilience.

Aside from the demands in clinical practice, there is also a need to develop resilience in your personal life and maybe throughout a course of study undertaken as part of your continuing professional development (CPD). One of the most misunderstood beliefs about resilience is that people are born resilient and that this cannot be changed or altered in any way. The importance of developing resilience cannot be underestimated as it has been shown to affect our health, emotional wellbeing, academic achievement, and relationships (Craig 2019). Resilience can in fact be learned and like other interpersonal communication skills such as assertiveness it can be practised, refined, and become part of your everyday life. However, before we start to think about how this can be done, it is important to define what is meant by resilience and what it 'looks' like.

WHAT IS RESILIENCE?

There is an abundance of definitions of resilience in the literature, some of which focus on the ability of an individual to overcome or recover from stress/trauma, others focus on a more positive aspect such as positive responses to events and cultivating effective coping strategies. Whichever perspective is taken, the consensus is that the development of resilience enables an individual to cope more effectively with sustained levels of stress

TABLE 3.1   Defining resilience.

Resilience is:	Resilience is not:
Ability to bounce back – not being afraid to make mistakes and have the confidence to act and manage situations	Denying/avoiding negative emotions
Being able to express emotions – being able to accept and acknowledge a range of difficult mentions. They do not view any emotion such as anxiety or sadness as a failing or weakness.	Bottling things up, pretending everything is fine
Not being afraid to ask for help and building support networks which are effectively used	Refusing to ask for help
Accepting that everything is not okay and that something(s) may need to change	Just getting on with it

and equips them to move forward more effectively. Below are two personal favourite definitions:

"the ability of an individual to respond positively and consistently to adversity, using effective coping strategies."

—Hunter and Warren 2014

"The capacity of individuals to navigate their way to ... resources ..., and ... individually and collectively to negotiate them ...."

—Ungar 2008

These not only highlight an individual's ability to cope, but also focus on their capacity to seek out and use the available resources to overcome adversity. This is particularly relevant to student radiographers, but also newly qualified practitioners during early transition and those moving into new professional roles.

Aspects of resilience are defined in Table 3.1.

THE IMPORTANCE AND ROLE OF SELF-AWARENESS

Before moving on to consider how you can develop and enhance your resilience, it is important to have an understanding of where you are now.

By completing the activity below, you will be able to identify how resilient you currently are, and it will give you a starting point to work from. Do not worry if you have a low score, the latter part of this chapter will help you to understand why and suggest ways in which you can develop your resilience.

ACTIVITY 3.2

Complete the abbreviated version of the Nicholson McBride Resilience questionnaire (NMRQ) at `https://www.nhsggc.org.uk/media/262884/resilience-questionnaire-fillable.pdf`.

Calculate your results:

80% or higher – very resilient!!

65–80% – better than most

50–65% – slow, but adequate

40–50% – you're struggling

40% or under – seek help!

After reading the descriptors, what are your initial thoughts, are you results what you expected?

THE SKILLS OF RESILIENCE, THE GROWTH MINDSET, AND THE INTERNAL LOCUS OF CONTROL

Remember, resilience can be learnt. When an individual chooses to see mistakes, difficulty, and challenges as an opportunity to learn, they are in a much better position to deal with these and therefore develop resilience. For example, if you can resist the urge to be concerned about looking 'stupid' you are more likely to ask questions, take feedback onboard, and learn more. This is true in all walks of life and in all situations.

The Growth Mindset (Figure 3.1) helps us to understand how our mindset can affect the way in which we approach situations. If you look at the fixed mindset, there is a belief that we are unable to change, learn, and grow from situations and that failure is final, whereas someone with a growth mindset will view failure as an opportunity to grow and enjoy challenges and to try new things. With this in mind, those with a fixed mindset will tend to be less resilient and will be unable to see how they can develop resilience by practice,

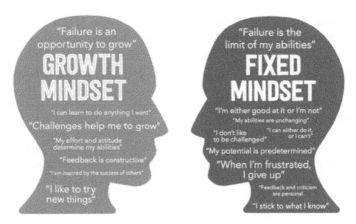

FIGURE 3.1   The growth mindset.

however those with a growth mindset will tend to be more resilient and open to ways in which they can develop their resilience even further. Looking at Figure 3.1 are you able to identify yourself as either of the mindsets?

Your mindset links strongly to the Locus of Control, which refers to how much a person feels that they can control their own behaviour. Rotter (1954) defines two aspects: Internal Locus of Control and External Locus of Control. Those with a high Internal Locus of Personal Control are more likely to take responsibility for the way that they behave as they have a good level of personal control over their behaviour (growth mindset). In contrast those who have an External Locus of Control, believe that their behaviour is because of external influences or luck (fixed mindset).

Individuals with a High Internal Locus of Control tend to be confident that they are able to handle and shape their own life whereas those with a Low External Locus of Control feel that their life is constrained by outside factors which they are unable to control. Referring back to Table 3.1 and Figure 3.1, links to both the growth mindset and aspects of resilience can be made.

DEVELOPING AND MAINTAINING YOUR RESILIENCE

If you have a Growth Mindset and a High Internal Locus of Control you will already be thinking about how you can develop your resilience, especially in your workplace. There are three skills that underpin resilience: emotional regulation, self-compassion, and cognitive agility. Emotional regulation is the ability to monitor, recognise, and respond to our emotions. Being able to have

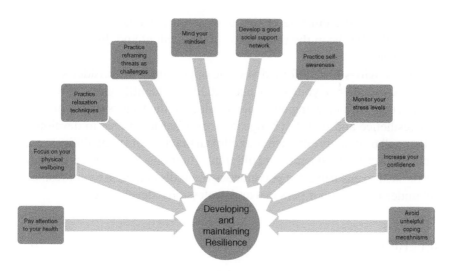

FIGURE 3.2 Developing resilience. Source: Adapted from Waters (2021).

an internal dialogue, pause, and think before responding to certain situations, especially when it causes a negative feeling inside is a sign of strong emotional regulation. It is when you solve problems by logical thought and not an emotional reaction. Self-compassion is about paying attention to ourselves, being kind, mindful, and forgiving. The aim is to reduce self-criticism and allow recognition of disappointment, sadness, and insecurity as normal. It is an acceptance of these as part of everyday life and then to have the ability to move on. Finally, cognitive agility involves recognising when thinking about a situation from one perspective has a negative impact on us. It helps us to focus on all possible aspects of a situation and to see other people's viewpoints. This will allow you to then discuss the situation in a measured and balanced way.

According to Waters (2021), there are also eight other ways in which you can develop your resilience which are summarised in Figure 3.2.

SUMMARY

In this chapter we have explored the concept and importance of resilience when working within a healthcare environment. It would be remiss not to mention the responsibility of the organisation to protect and support their employees and there is certainly more work to be done by the NHS in this area. However, the purpose of this book is on personal development and therefore this has been the main focus of the content and discussion within this chapter.

The activities have afforded you the opportunity to consider situations which may challenge your resilience and to also identify your current level of resilience. By increasing an understanding of the factors which influence your resilience and how to change your mindset to be able to develop this further will ultimately enhance your clinical practice and your ability to effectively communicate in a range of different situations. Resilience is not inherited or fixed so ensuring that you practice the skills to increase your resilience will underpin both your personal and professional development.

REFERENCES

Borras, J.M., Lievens, Y., Barton, M. et al. (2016). How many new cancer patients in Europe will require radiotherapy by 2025? An ESTRO-HERO analysis. *Radiotherapy and Oncology* 119 (1): 5–11. https://doi.org/10.1016/j.radonc.2016.02.016. Epub 2016 Feb 24. PMID: 26922487.

Craig, H. (2019). Resilience in the workplace: how to be more resilient at work. https://positivepsychology.com/resilience-in-the-workplace (accessed 20 February 2023).

Hunter, B. and Warren, L.E. (2014). Midwives' experiences of workplace resilience. *Midwifery* (30): 8. https://doi.org/10.1016/j.midw.2014.03.010/.

Mann, S. (2005). A health-care model of emotional labour: an evaluation of the literature and development of a model. *Journal of Health Organization and Management* 19 (4/5): 304–317. https://doi.org/10.1108/14777260510615369.

McAllister, M. and McKinnon, J. (2009). The importance of teaching and learning in the health disciplines: a critical review of the literature. *Nurse Education Today* (29): 371–379.

NHS Confederation (2014). *The 2015 Challenge Declaration*. London: NHS Confederation.

Rotter, J.B. (1954). *Social Learning and Clinical Psychology*. New York: Prentice-Hall.

Skovolt, T. (2001). *The Resilient Practitioner*. Boston: Allyn and Bacon.

Ungar, M. (2008). Resilience across cultures. *British Journal of Social Work* 38 (2): 218–235.

Waters, S. (2021). Why building resilience is a top skill for the workplace. https://www.betterup.com/blog/how-to-build-resilience-why-resilience-is-a-top-skill-for-the-workplace (accessed 20 February 2023).

Wieclaw, J., Agerbo, E., Mortensen, P., and Bonde, J. (2006). Risk of affective and stress related disorders among employees in human service professions. *Occupational and Environmental Medicine* 63: 314–319.

CHAPTER 4

What Is Compassion?

Amy Hancock, Jane Gooch, and Jill Bleiker

Compassion is one of those words that everyone thinks means the same thing, but research shows that what patients see as compassion tends to differ from that of radiographers and students (Bleiker 2020; Taylor 2020). For example, patients see compassion in terms of behaviours and expressions that are visible or observable, such as noticing that a patient is cold or uncomfortable and fetching a blanket or pillow. Radiographers and students did mention these when asked, but believed they were more akin to acts of general kindness, seeing compassion as more specific actions they could take, for example minimising the duration of the procedure so that the patient was spending the shortest possible amount of time in discomfort. Patients, on the other hand, saw this as efficiency, proficiency, or professionalism, but not compassion.

Quite often people use other words that, for them, mean the same as compassion. In other words, not everyone agrees on exactly what they mean when they talk about compassion. Below you can see some examples of what people in the research conducted for this book say when they try to define or describe compassion.

WHAT IS COMPASSION?

Both diagnostic and therapeutic radiographers and student radiographers, as well as patients and carers used words like empathy, sympathy, understanding, and caring when describing compassion:

Person-centred Care in Radiography: Skills for Providing Effective Patient Care, First Edition.
Ruth M. Strudwick, Jane M. Harvey-Lloyd, Jill Bleiker, Jane Gooch, Amy Hancock,
Emma Hyde, and Ann Newton-Hughes.
© 2024 John Wiley & Sons Ltd. Published 2024 by John Wiley & Sons Ltd.

"I almost feel that compassion and empathy are kind of interchangeable in some ways. When I think of using the word compassionate in the sort of sentences I was using I could easily switch it out for empathise or empathy."

—Student therapeutic radiographer

"I do think that they need to use the word empathy in here because empathy is part of compassion. If you've got empathy with that person you can become compassionate towards them by understanding what they're going through. That makes it easy to be compassionate whereas if you don't understand how that person's feeling, how can you possibly be compassionate?"

—Diagnostic radiography patient

"I think it's kind of being kind to people and kind of sympathy at the same time and empathy."

—Student therapeutic radiographer

"I see compassion as being more having an understanding of what someone's going through and caring about it."

—Diagnostic radiography patient

We could just leave it at that and settle for compassion as being 'something a bit like empathy' or sympathy. From listening to our patients though, it is clear that they feel it is important for radiographers to understand what compassion is and to demonstrate how it is different from other similar concepts as this will affect how they receive and interpret it.

"I see sympathy as much, a bit more, poor you, as opposed to compassion…which isn't necessarily what you want when you're undergoing something: you want someone that's not necessarily been through the same thing as you but that gives the impression that they understand what you're going through even if they actually don't."

—Diagnostic radiography patient

"I see compassion as quite a positive thing and someone would display compassion. But the definition here is quite negative in terms of the words that were used like pity and suffering and misfortune."

—Therapeutic radiography patient

" ... to me compassion is a very personal thing because one person's compassion is another person's fussing, isn't it?"

—Diagnostic radiography patient

"I just think, to be compassionate means to sort of identify that you are struggling or something like that but, I wouldn't want pity."

—Therapeutic radiography patient

So, we really do need to tease out these concepts in order to give the most appropriate care to each individual patient – the very definition of 'person-centred care'.

SO, WHAT IS EMPATHY THEN?

We have identified that empathy is a word that is often used when trying to define or explain the meaning of compassion. As part of any health care professional training, the backbone of your education will be formed of anatomical and medical knowledge, as well as specific technical and practical skills. However, the sometimes-called 'softer' emotion-based skills of empathy and compassion used as part of our everyday practice when we communicate and interact with patients can sometimes be overlooked (Taylor et al. 2021). However, these skills are an equally important component and one of the ways we try to think about how patients or others might feel is through the use of reflection and reflective practice (Schon 1984). We sometimes use manikin patients to practise our positioning and technique skills, but how realistic is that when you are trying to work out how the patient might be feeling? Would you even talk to the manikin or are you too busy concentrating on their body part?

If empathy is something like an affinity with another person, or an appreciation of them, and that person happens to be the patient currently in your care, how do we go about understanding what they are going through without having a long, in-depth (and time-consuming) conversation with them? Firstly, they may not want to share their innermost feelings with you, and secondly you do not have time anyway, so what can you do to get some rapport going? Research suggests that the first brief moment you interact with the patient is central to their experience in your care (Taylor et al. 2017; Bleiker 2020). How you introduce yourself and create that fleeting relationship with the patient is crucial; you may find out quite a lot in those few minutes which will help you empathise with them and make an appraisal of the appropriateness of compassionate gestures and acts.

Reflective Exercise

What comes to mind when you think about the word 'Compassion'?

Spend a few moments and either come up with words, ideas, or perhaps images which you would use to explain it to someone else.

Now think about what comes to mind when you think about the word 'Empathy'? Spend a few moments and either come up with words, ideas, or perhaps images which you would use to explain it to someone else.

Now think about them both; what do you think are the differences between the two concepts?

DEFINING CHARACTERISTICS OF COMPASSION

Research shows that compassion within a healthcare setting is comprised of five defining attributes or characteristics (Taylor et al. 2017):

1. Recognition: Cognitive recognition (noticing and mentally processing) another's adverse circumstances, with concern for their physical, psychological or emotional well-being.
2. Connection: Personal connection with another based on automatic, authentic and genuine thought.
3. Altruistic desire: A humane wish to aid another.
4. Humanistic response: Human-centred, person-to-person, understanding of what it is to be human.
5. Action: Undertaking of an act or responsive behaviour.

Although these occur sequentially and each attribute needs to occur, the individual who is to display compassion may need to move between the attributes depending on the situation. Figure 4.1 shows the defining attributes or characteristics of compassion.

As you can see in Figure 4.1, the first two of the five defining characteristics of compassion are Recognition, and Connection. *Recognising* your patient's adverse circumstances: not just their physical, but their psychological or emotional state too, and *Connecting* with them by looking

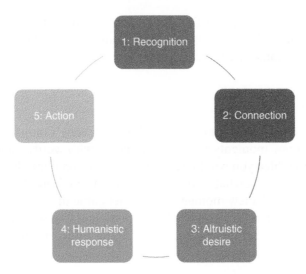

FIGURE 4.1   Defining attributes of compassion in healthcare (Taylor et al. 2017).

at their face, and into their eyes. Uncomfortable for both of you if it turns into staring, but a glance will tell you if they seem relaxed or tense; are they returning your welcoming smile? Or are they stony faced? Are they walking with ease, or is their face twisted in pain? Look for the *non-verbal* cues that give clues to what is going on in the minds and bodies of your patients. This may or may not trigger feelings in you of sympathy or even pity perhaps, but it has the added benefit of giving you clues as to how well your patient is going to be able to co-operate with the procedure, how easily they will be able to get into and hold the positions needed for accurate imaging or treatment. Are they breathing heavily? That will affect how well they will be able to hold their breath for you, and if you *recognise* that it might be difficult for them, then hey presto – you are *empathising* with them!

Your patient may not be displaying any signs that they are suffering discomfort or distress, or, as we have seen when thinking about compassion, they may not *want* expressions of sympathy or pity rather a recognition or acknowledgement of the discomfort of the examination or procedure they are about to undergo:

"I didn't want a hug and a 'you okay?' but it would just have been an acknowledgement that 'this is painful' would have had me better prepared."

—Diagnostic radiography patient

"I'd rather competence and respect if I was a patient, not compassion; that can easily resemble pity."

—Diagnostic radiographer

Reflective Exercise

Think about all the non-verbal cues you could look for that would give you clues as to the 'hidden' thoughts and feelings your patient could be experiencing whilst in your care.

WHY SHOULD RADIOGRAPHERS BE COMPASSIONATE?

The third characteristic, *Altruistic Desire* or the 'motivation' to be compassionate provides us with the opportunity to consider why we should be compassionate to our patients. From a professional perspective in the United Kingdom we need to meet the standards required for professional registration by practising in compliance with the Society and College of Radiographers (SCoR) Code of Professional Conduct (Society and College of Radiographers 2013) and the Health and Care Professions Council (HCPC) Standards of Proficiency (Health and Care Professions Council 2013). During radiographic imaging and treatment, we are required to 'provide the best compassionate care for patients based on up-to-date evidence' (Society and College of Radiographers 2013) and 'understand the need to act in the best interests of service users at all times' (Health and Care Professions Council 2013). A failure to be motivated to exercise compassion with our patients during their diagnostic imaging or radiotherapy procedure could mean that we are not practising in accordance with the standards required for professional registration. Although professionally important, it is also essential that we reflect upon and consider to whom our compassion is being directed; the answer is the human beings who are our patients as we practice our professions. Not only are we responsible for the management of care and services for a wide range of people who attend our departments for radiographic or therapeutic procedures, each requiring our input to support them in their medical pathway, but we also hold their emotional welfare in our hands as we image or treat them. The literature demonstrates how being compassionate has positive consequences for both patient and practitioner, illustrating the positivity of compassion within our person-centred interactions (Taylor et al. 2017) (Figure 4.2).

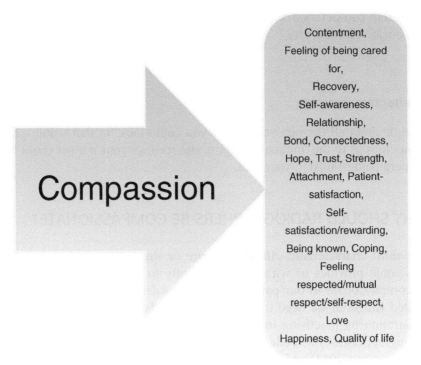

Contentment,
Feeling of being cared
for,
Recovery,
Self-awareness,
Relationship,
Bond, Connectedness,
Hope, Trust, Strength,
Attachment, Patient-
satisfaction,
Self-
satisfaction/rewarding,
Being known, Coping,
Feeling
respected/mutual
respect/self-respect,
Love
Happiness, Quality of life

FIGURE 4.2   Consequences of compassion (Taylor et al. 2017).

Reflective Exercise

Think about a time when you have been compassionate and ask yourself;
    Why did you decide to be compassionate, how did it make you feel,
how did the patient (or other person) react?

In Chapter 7, we will look at the characteristics *Humanistic Response* and *Action* which are the practical steps you can take to take care of patients' psychological and emotional welfare during diagnostic imaging or therapy treatment. To close this chapter, we will use the following scenarios taken from real patient experiences to reflect on and cement your understanding of compassion and its relationship with, in particular, empathy, but also the other closely associated concepts. Read the scenarios and consider how the radiographer's actions and behaviours illustrated relate to the defining attributes outlined above, and to compassion and empathy more generally.

What went well, and what not so well? What else, if anything, could the radiographers in these scenarios have done?

Scenario 4.1

Frank was attending his weekly review with the specialist therapeutic radiographer as part of his radiotherapy treatment for prostate cancer. He'd been worried for some time about problems he was experiencing with his erection and had wanted to ask someone but had felt too embarrassed. His wife had told him that he must speak to someone at his next appointment as it was becoming a problem for them as a couple. Towards the end of his review the radiographer asked him if there was anything else she could help him with. Frank told her about the problems he and his wife were experiencing when they tried to have intercourse, to which she replied that it was just an effect of his diagnosis and the radiotherapy treatment. Frank expressed that he knew this, but his original consultant had said there were some options and maybe some medication he could take. Reluctantly the radiographer nodded and replied this was not her area and so would go and ask a colleague for some advice. The radiographer exited the room into the main waiting area leaving Frank sat alone with the door open. Whilst Frank was waiting, he could hear laughter, listening in he heard his specialist radiographer saying (laughing)… "I know, tell me about it and it his age it…(laughter), yeah good point I will tell him to Google it, there will be plenty of stuff on the internet for that kind of thing… well yeah, I suppose whatever floats your boat" (laughter).

Scenario 4.2

Claire said: "I think it was last year when I had a barium follow through. I told the radiographer that I could have difficulty drinking this stuff and the likelihood is that I would be sick. "No, you'll be fine, no problem, don't worry about it" she said, and I said, "well, you've been told." You're expected to sit in the corridor and take it, there's nowhere you can go, no privacy or anything, and I said, "I can't drink this in a busy corridor with people sitting watching, it's not right." And she said, "well, I'm sorry, there's nowhere else" and she directed me to the disabled toilet and I took it in there. This happens today, this is common practice. You drink the stuff where they give it to you in a corridor. I'm surprised they don't give you barium enemas in the corridor as well."

Scenario 4.3

Clive, a therapeutic radiographer for 20 years, was chatting with a 19-year-old patient called John who was about to start radical radiotherapy for testicular cancer. John was telling him that he had already had the tumour and his left testicle removed and how he had to make the difficult decision as to whether to have his sperm frozen or not before he started radiotherapy. John told Clive that it has sparked him and his girlfriend to think about their futures together and they had decided to get married. He confessed he was worried and kept on stressing over whether the sperm banking process may not have worked and that he was worried how his fiancée would take the news if this was the case. Clive sat and listened to the young man's fears, ensuring that he knew he was there for him to talk to. Clive fully understood how John was feeling; not only had he treated many patients like John over his professional career, but when Clive himself was 22 he had received the same diagnosis so knew what John must have been going through.

Scenario 4.4

Jane attended for a diagnostic X-ray examination of a painful elbow that had been going on for several months. Upon entering the X-ray room, the radiographer introduced herself to Jane by name and then asked her about her particular problem. The radiographer said things like "That is a bit unusual, how long have you been suffering from this?" and "are you hoping to get some results from this?" She followed this with an explanation of what she was about to do and how she was going to do it. Jane was impressed with the interaction, and the fact that the radiographer asked her why she was there, and what she expected from it.

Scenario 4.5

Ron attended for an X-ray examination of the hip he recently had replaced. He described his feelings having only just had the surgery saying: "that was two days after the hip replacement and it was still a... well I'm fairly bullish about things but it was still a relatively nervous time, I had no expectation or understanding

really apart from reading a few pamphlets which doesn't give you the depth".
The radiographer revealed that she had a close relative who had had a hip oper-
ation relatively recently and Ron remarked that although it was "just a bit of
pleasant conversation drawing parallels" it was nevertheless "a nice softener –
it was not necessary, just a nice touch. Her approach was pretty much spot on as
in the empathy – drawing parallels with previous cases and positive outcomes
just generally putting me at ease, so the fact that she could relate stories, a story
of a relative who had had a good outcome it all sort of helped with going in the
right direction."

REFERENCES

Bleiker, J. (2020). An inquiry into compassion in diagnostic radiography. Unpublished thesis.

Health and Care Professions Council (2013). Standards of proficiency for radiographers. Radiographers.

Schon, D.A. (1984). *The Reflective Practitioner: How Professionals Think In Action*, 1e. Basic Books.

Society and College of Radiographers (2013). Code of professional conduct.

Taylor, A. (2020). Defining compassion and compassionate behaviour in radiotherapy. Unpublished thesis.

Taylor, A., Hodgson, D., Gee, M., and Collins, K. (2017). Compassion in Healthcare: a concept analysis. *Journal of Radiotherapy in Practice* 16: 350–360. https://doi.org/10.1017/S1460396917000322.

Taylor, A., Bleiker, J., and Hodgson, D. (2021). Compassionate communication: keeping patients at the heart of practice in an advancing radiographic workforce. *Radiography* 27: S43–S49.

CHAPTER 5

Pain and Suffering

Ann Newton-Hughes, Amy Hancock, and Jill Bleiker

The notion of suffering has been found in radiography research to be an interesting one; it might interest you to know that the Latin word for suffering is '*passion*' and that 'com-passion' means 'to *suffer with*' (OED, n.d.) someone. Even the term 'patient' means 'one who suffers' (OED, n.d.), although patients in one study (Bleiker 2020) did not like to be thought of as suffering:

"but then this person came along and said, 'do you suffer with a low heart rate?' and I said, 'I don't suffer at all.' It was just the wrong choice of word"

—Diagnostic radiography patient

During the interview, the patient didn't explain why she didn't like the choice of word; what do you think might have been behind her comment? The thoughts of this patient may give you some ideas:

"I see compassion as quite a positive thing, and someone would display compassion. But the definition here is quite negative in terms of the words that were used like pity and suffering and misfortune"

—Therapeutic radiography patient

This chapter is concerned with what is meant by pain and suffering, together with perceptions around them such as that seen in the examples above. How pain and suffering factor in the specific context of your radiographic professional practice will also be discussed.

Person-centred Care in Radiography: Skills for Providing Effective Patient Care, First Edition.
Ruth M. Strudwick, Jane M. Harvey-Lloyd, Jill Bleiker, Jane Gooch, Amy Hancock,
Emma Hyde, and Ann Newton-Hughes.
© 2024 John Wiley & Sons Ltd. Published 2024 by John Wiley & Sons Ltd.

PAIN AND SUFFERING: SUBTLE DIFFERENCES

Pain is a complex mix of nerve signal, emotion, and processing within the brain. It can be categorised in three ways (The British Pain Society, n.d.):

- Acute – a short term warning pain that provokes action i.e. resting if you have broken a limb.
- Chronic – sometimes has no currently useful purpose but it can affect the ability to work, sleep and enjoy life.
- Intermittent – such as a toothache or back ache.

As radiographers we will encounter patients experiencing all these types of pain. Pain is unpleasant and it can be physically, mentally, and emotionally difficult for our patients to manage on top of everything else that is going on in their lives. Emotions such as anger, depression, and anxiety can exacerbate perceptions of pain (Swift 2018) and it is therefore important that as radiographers we bear this in mind whilst imaging or treating patients. It is important to be aware of the effects of pain, for example, someone in chronic pain may also be sleep deprived and perhaps depressed, and this may account for a patient's behaviour (such as a lack of cooperation) even though there appears to be no obvious explanation at first (Wilson et al. 2002).

Suffering on the other hand is the *experiencing* of pain, distress, or hardship and, like pain itself can be physical, psychological, or emotional (Hudson 2012). It can be caused by such events as illness, injury, loss, or even the anticipation of any of these. Suffering can cause physical and psychological responses including effects on the cardiovascular, endocrine, gastrointestinal, urinary, and immune systems alongside musculoskeletal changes which may include muscle stiffness and shaking, any of which can impact on patient positioning for imaging or therapy. Psychological responses can include, stress, anger, feeling misunderstood, depression, and anxiety (Mager, n.d.) and radiographers will need to understand these responses alongside the physical manifestations of the patient's suffering.

PERCEPTIONS OF PAIN AND SUFFERING

Perceptions of pain and suffering differ widely between individuals and can vary along the lines of age (Olson 2015), gender (Bullock 2018), and culture (Peacock and Patel 2008) as well as other factors such as upbringing and social influences (Sharma et al. 2018). Patients may also be reluctant to show, express, or report pain; in one doctoral study, reasons for hiding feelings and emotions included a desire to co-operate in order to expedite (speed up) the procedure, perceived generational norms, or stoicism (Bleiker 2020). We will detail some examples but do bear in mind that when it comes to your assessment of a patient's suffering this should be made on a case-by-case basis and that the worst thing you could do is to generalise or in any way 'play down' a patient's experience; that would be to diminish them as well as their suffering.

Reflective Exercise

Current research does not show a consistent link between increasing age and pain perception; in one study 60–75% of people over the age of 65 reported experiencing persistent pain (Tsang et al. 2008), whereas those over 85 reported less pain (Helme and Gibson 2001). Do you think that elderly patients are experiencing less pain or under reporting it? Do people become more stoical as they get older, or do they perhaps get used to a greater level of pain? Is it something to do with how you are brought up (i.e. the values instilled from childhood)? Or maybe it is to do with the norms for your particular generation? How would that affect how you interact with and care for this age group? You can take some clues from the quotes below (Bleiker 2020):

" ... you don't want a fuss, so you quite often ... yes, I have laid there in the most uncomfortable position sometimes, not wanting to say, 'have you got a pillow or two?"

—Diagnostic radiography patient

"It's not so much these days but in my mother's generation to show emotion, to show distress was not, was a thing you didn't do. It's stiff upper lip and ... "

—Diagnostic radiography patient

Interviewer: " ... and I imagine you were trying to be stoical and brave and ...

Respondent: I was, absolutely, yes. I always try and be polite to people at least ... "

—Diagnostic radiography patient

The patient in the following example was not especially elderly but had been in pain for quite some time. Can you see the clue in what they said as to why they may not have revealed just how much pain they were experiencing?

"at the time I went in for that appointment, I was in the process . . . I'd been living with the pain for a while and going to see the consultant or going to see the radiographer . . . was all part of steps that I had to take before the right diagnosis to be achieved and so I wasn't squirming, 'oh, that hurts,' or so I didn't really do anything that I would have thought evoked anybody to go, 'are you alright, dear?' kind of thing. I'm a little bit, kind of, deal with it and so I probably wouldn't have given any signals that I needed emotional support or reassurance or anything like that but I think I probably would have come over as a fairly confident person . . . "

—Diagnostic radiography patient

In the example above the patient stated that *"I'm a little bit, kind of, deal with it"* suggesting subtle differences in even perhaps a patient's personality may be in play. The example also shows that differences exist in the expression of emotions around pain and suffering with sometimes high, and what appear to be dramatic outbursts from some patients whilst others supress, or at least attempt to supress their feelings of suffering. Make sure to look at your patient's face when positioning them for imaging or treatment and not just at the body part you are focussed on, as a great deal can be read and interpreted from facial expressions. Take care though to check in with your patient, as a grimace can be misinterpreted as anger or aggression instead of pain. Also watch your patient's posture and the way they move, as more clues can be gained from these non-verbal cues as this student radiographer observed (Bleiker 2020):

"If you call from the waiting room and just depending on how they stand up for a start you can like . . . yeah . . . start like treating them differently . . . "

—Student diagnostic radiographer

What is clear is that perceptions of, and reactions to pain and suffering differ widely between individuals. Giving person-centred care means that in the same way that we respect the values of our patients we need to respect and act appropriately for the pain the patient is experiencing, ensuring that we adapt our communication to show that we understand their suffering. This will undoubtedly mean that we need to put aside our own understanding of pain levels and behaviour. These examples from the authors' doctoral research show how you might adapt your communication and professional practice in supporting your patients (Bleiker 2020; Taylor 2020):

"She ran through it all first which was really good 'cos then I knew and then I could say 'actually when you do that, I'm gonna find that painful' so then she remembered"

—Diagnostic radiography patient

"I get migraines and people say have you got a headache? No; I've got a migraine. It's different. You know? But because it's lack of understanding that sometimes brings about lack of compassion"

—Therapeutic radiography patient

"I didn't want a hug and a 'you okay?' but … an acknowledgement that 'this is painful' would have had me better prepared [for the discomfort of the examination]"

—Diagnostic radiography patient

"So, when I approached her [the patient] she started crying. So, I asked her, and she said no it's too painful, I don't know what to do about it, I feel like I want to just stop this [the radiotherapy] because it is not working for me. I said to her, do you want to talk to someone, or do you want us to do anything for you? She was like, I just want a chat, I just want to chat to someone, because she felt like we didn't give her enough time, you know, for her to explain what she was going through"

—Student therapeutic radiographer

As you can see, the aim is not necessarily to relieve the pain, that is often not possible, but to relieve the suffering associated with it – as surely an act of compassion as relieving the pain itself.

ATTITUDES TO PAIN AND SUFFERING

Attitudes to suffering vary widely and opinions can be formed based on whether the suffering of others is perceived as avoidable or deserved. Some people will find it difficult to empathise with those who they believe have caused their own suffering (Gibb et al. 2010).

Reflective Exercise

Consider the relevant scenario for your profession:

Diagnostic: Your patient has presented with pain and swelling over the outside of their hand. The request form reads 'query fracture of the head of the fifth metacarpal'. You have learned that by far the most common way of sustaining this injury is from punching something or someone. The patient has a shaved head and numerous tattoos visible and appears sullen and unwilling to communicate with you.

Therapeutic: Your patient arrives for head and neck radiotherapy complaining of severe pain in their throat when trying to swallow fluids. During your interaction you can smell alcohol strongly on their breath.

Is compassion a feeling that arises within you at the plight of your patient?

As radiographers we will encounter patients experiencing differing types of pain and suffering and our professional code of conduct requires that we empathise with them without judgement (HCPC 2013). We must also be aware of the different ways in which people will express their pain so that we do not make assumptions and underestimate the level of pain the patient is experiencing.

It is important that as professionals we consider how patients are trying to deal with the psychological and physical effects of their pain or diagnosis, and to remember that wider issues such as work, family, and financial matters might also be causing suffering. Smoking, for example is widely cited as a coping mechanism for dealing with stress (Wells et al. 2017). It is important, but sometimes difficult not to judge but instead realise that patients bring these issues with them as well as the clinical ones with which they present, and we should use that understanding in our interaction.

In order to practise with understanding and empathy it is also important as professionals that we manage our own wellbeing, including our own physical and mental health. Our professional and governing bodies recognise this in our codes of conduct as it is a requirement to seek help when needed. Support is available for radiographers through our employers and the Society and College of Radiographers initiatives such as the 'Radiate' campaign (Society of Radiographers Radiate: Wellbeing Hub, n.d.). Advice can also be found in Chapter 3 which discussed resilience.

HOW IS PAIN MEASURED?

It is widely accepted that self-reporting is the most accurate measure of pain level for cognitively able patients and one-dimensional pain scales are often used to give a numerical value to the level of pain experienced by the patient to help us get some idea of their suffering (Dalton and McNaull 1998). These provide an indication of the level of pain experienced by the patient at the time the measure was taken but are seldom used when imaging or treating patients. There are however limitations to these, can you think what they might be? Rather than using a pain scale radiographers may be able to form their own assessment of the level of pain and suffering of the patient based on a variety of clues provided (Newton-Hughes 2015). In any case, patients should be able to feel that their radiographer has listened to them and respects their perceptions of what they are enduring in that moment, so the patient should be consulted on how best they can achieve the positions required for imaging or treatment and helped or encouraged to achieve this, however long it might take over and above the expected time for the examination or procedure.

GIVING PERSON-CENTRED CARE TO PATIENTS IN PAIN AND SUFFERING IN IMAGING EXAMINATIONS AND RADIOTHERAPY TREATMENTS

The ways we can support and care for our patients are many and varied. To start with, the radiographer can review the prior information available to them about the patient. For patients undergoing medical imaging, this information will come from the imaging request and any previous images seen on the Picture Archiving and Communications System (PACS), whereas for therapy patients, the radiographer will have access to the patient notes and their referral form. You can also consider informal cues, for example the mode of transport used by the patient to get to the department, or the clinical history given by the patient whilst talking to them prior to starting the examination or treatment to gain an understanding of the level of pain or discomfort being experienced (Newton-Hughes and Robinson 2013). It is important to help support the patient to reduce the pain experienced, and although we may not be able to get the pain under control, if we can help them feel calmer and less upset that will help us achieve our aims of accurate imaging or treatment. Prior to starting their radiotherapy, patients may have undergone surgery and could still be affected by the pain and discomfort associated with this. If inoperable the tumour itself can be a cause of pain and those patients receiving palliative therapy for metastatic disease will in general be affected by pain in the site of secondary tumours, (colloquially known as 'mets', short for metastases) for example in their bones, brain or spine.

Even before you start your interaction with the patient you can get hints from such clues as whether and how they are walking, perhaps hesitantly, awkwardly, or with the help of a stick, or are unable to walk at all and present to you on a chair or trolley. Take the opportunity to assess your patient's movement, body language, facial expression and speech to give an indication of the level of pain they are experiencing (Newton-Hughes and Robinson 2013). Consider also other health conditions the patient might be suffering which could exacerbate any pain they are experiencing. You could also question the patient in relation to their ability to move and position for the examination or treatment. Patients in pain may struggle to comply with the instructions we give before and during the examination or treatment and we need to be prepared to adapt both how we communicate with our patient as well as our radiographic or positioning technique (Newton-Hughes 2015). As the interaction progresses you can continue to use communication and observation to evaluate the patient, paying particular attention to verbal and non-verbal expressions of pain (Newton-Hughes and Robinson 2013).

Pain can be caused or exacerbated by the positioning we use for imaging or treatment. Whilst some adaptation of techniques can be used to minimise the impact in diagnostic imaging, this is more challenging in radiotherapy due to the necessity to keep the patient immobilized for up to 30 minutes. Subsequently, causing pain can be unavoidable and has been shown to be distressing for the patient, particularly if the radiographer lacks understanding or empathy and is focussed only on the radiographic task (Bleiker 2020):

"they [the radiographer] said, 'you need to get it straight' [the patient was referring to their fractured elbow] I said, 'I can't get it straight, any straighter than that and I'm in agony.' With that a senior radiographer come in and said, 'what's all the noise?' They said, 'this patient is being obstructive.' So he said, 'what seems to be the problem?' I said, 'I fell on my elbow and I cannot get my elbow out straight,' I said"

—Diagnostic radiography patient

During radiotherapy any existing pain suffered by the patient may be exacerbated by their position and need for immobilisation on the treatment couch. The treatment couch is hard and uncushioned, due to the need to keep the patient in a fixed position without any rotation or sinking into the couch. Patients with bone metastases can be in excruciating pain and can find positioning on the table particularly uncomfortable (NHS 2020).

Caring for the patient in pain requires skilful communication using non-verbal cues such as eye contact to signal empathy and understanding, gentle handling, and, perhaps most difficult of all for the novice practitioner, conveying confidence to the patient that they are in safe and competent hands. This communication skill is tacitly acquired with experience and through observation of more experienced colleagues. Student radiographers express initial concern related to the pain caused by positioning patients but accept that this is often a requirement of the role.

After an examination, diagnostic radiographers are often unaware of potential after-effects as patients' visits to imaging are short and the radiographer is unlikely to know if a patient undergoes a 'flare up' of their condition or prolonged pain after experiencing an imaging examination. Similarly, unless involved in a role which includes patient follow-up, therapeutic radiographers will not be privy to some of the acute and to the main chronic side effects of radiotherapy. Some imaging examinations are invasive, i.e. involve punctures or incisions and may have painful aftereffects. In diagnostic imaging scant attention is paid to the level of pain following an invasive procedure; in these cases, after care is provided to the patient, but this may be provided by the department nurse. In radiotherapy practice attention is paid to the side effects the patient is currently experiencing and medications are prescribed to help reduce the pain and discomfort caused by these. Therapeutic radiographers can also be involved with referring patients to specialists.

The cumulative build-up of radiation dose during radiotherapy will mean patients can suffer increasing pain during and throughout the course of their treatment. Some invasive diagnostic procedures may impact on short term activities; for example, following an examination which requires the administration of barium sulphate contrast media (NHS 2022). After radiotherapy, internal and external side effects are inevitable, for example in areas where the skin rubs together such as under the fold of the breast or groin and can be very sore for weeks after the end of treatment. Similarly, any existing pain caused by metastatic disease or symptoms of the cancer can be worsened by the radiotherapy treatment. The memory of these experiences can linger, as our research revealed when interviewing and talking to patients who had undergone imaging and/or treatment, sometimes many years previously (Bleiker 2020; Taylor 2020).

Unfortunately, pressures of time and workload mean that some patients can be left feeling worse, both physically and mentally after their procedure (Bleiker 2020):

"I felt like there possibly wasn't the understanding that they'd just taken the plaster off and I feel like I'm going to die or someone's gonna hit me, that's....I'm... but you're frightened of someone going near it"

—Diagnostic radiography patient

"No warmth or understanding or that actually, 'dislocating your knee hurts like hell', and 'you're probably gonna be in pain'... "

—Diagnostic radiography patient

Radiographers do acknowledge that causing physical or mental suffering for the patient can induce a sense of guilt. This extends beyond simply hurting the patient in the course of the examination or treatment procedure as this radiographer tweeted somewhat ruefully, as indicated by the :- emoji (Bleiker 2020).

"I have definitely been guilty of cutting corners and not listening to patients when super busy :- "

—diagnostic radiographer

SUMMARY

This chapter has teased apart the variety of ways in which pain and suffering are experienced by patients. How a patient perceives, reacts, and behaves is therefore highly subjective and radiographers should strive to ensure that the care and support they offer to the patient is not influenced by judgmentalism or personal views and perceptions, but by a need to care with compassion whilst producing the best quality images or giving the most effective treatment possible.

LIST OF TOP TIPS TO ENSURE CARE FOR PATIENTS IN PAIN OR SUFFERING

1. LOOK for clues in patients' physical presentation including mode of transport (walking, chair, trolley), verbal and non-verbal cues.

2. SEARCH, more clues can be found from the clinical history, first on the request form, then by asking relevant and specific questions of the patient.

3. LISTEN to what the patient is telling you and ACT ON WHAT YOU HEAR. Do not focus just on the task of imaging or treatment, instead adapt what you might have planned to do, or say, in order to minimise their suffering, given that you may not be able to eliminate it completely.

4. REMEMBER that your patient's experience at your hands may stay with them for long after you and they have parted company. Some of the patients in the studies which inform this chapter were recalling memories from many years previously.

REFERENCES

Bleiker, J. (2020). An Inquiry into Compassion in Diagnostic Radiography. Unpublished thesis.

Bullock, J. (2018). *Pain Bias: The Health Inequality Rarely Discussed*. BBC Future.

Dalton, J.A. and McNaull, F. (1998). A call for standardizing the clinical rating of pain intensity using a 0 to 10 rating scale. *Cancer Nursing* 21: 46–49.

Gibb, S.J., Beautrais, A.L., and Surgenor, L.J. (2010). Health-care staff attitudes towards self-harm patients. *Australian and New Zealand Journal of Psychiatry.* 44 (8): 713–720. https://doi.org/10.3109/00048671003671015. PMID: 20636192.

HCPC (2013). Standards of proficiency for radiographers. https://www.hcpc-uk.org/standards/standards-of-proficiency/radiographers/ (accessed 20 February 2023).

Helme, R.D. and Gibson, S.J. (2001). The epidemiology of pain in elderly people. *Clinical Geriatric Medicine* 17: 417–431.

Hudson, W. (2012). Historicizing suffering. In: *Perspectives on Human Suffering* (ed. J. Malpas and N. Lickiss). Springer.

Mager, D. (n.d.). Pain is inevitable; suffering is optional. https://www.psychologytoday.com/us/blog/some-assembly-required/201401/pain-is-inevitable-suffering-is-optional (accessed 20 February 2023).

Newton-Hughes, A.M. (2015). An ethnographic study of radiographer problem solving and decision making in the trauma setting. DProf thesis. University of

Salford. https://core.ac.uk/download/pdf/42589686.pdf (accessed 20 February 2023).

Newton-Hughes, A., and Robinson, L. (2013). Radiographer Assessment of Patient Mobility in the Trauma Setting. E poster UKRC.

NHS (2020). Health A–Z side effects of radiotherapy. www.nhs.uk (accessed 20 February 2023).

NHS (2022). Health A–Z barium enema. www.nhs.uk (accessed 20 February 2023).

OED (n.d.). Oxford English dictionary (online). http://www.oed.com/ (accessed 20 February 2023).

Olson, K. (2015). Pain and aging. *Practical Pain Management* 15: 5.

Peacock, S. and Patel, S. (2008). Cultural influences on pain. *British Journal of Pain*. https://www.sor.org/events-programme/radiate.

Sharma, S., Abbott, J.H., and Jensen, M.P. (2018). Why clinicians should consider the role of culture in chronic pain. *Brazilian Journal of Physical Therapy* 22 (5): 345–346. https://doi.org/10.1016/j.bjpt.2018.07.002. PMID: 30126712; PMCID: PMC6157457.

Society of Radiographers Radiate: Wellbeing Hub (n.d.). https://www.sor.org/events-programme/radiate.

Swift, A. (2018). Understanding pain and the human body's response to it. *Nursing Times* 114 (3): 22–26.

Taylor, A. (2020). Defining Compassion and Compassionate Behaviour in Radiotherapy. Unpublished thesis.

The British Pain Society (n.d.). What is pain? https://www.britishpainsociety.org/about/what-is-pain/ (accessed 20 February 2023).

Tsang, A., Von Korff, M., Lee, S. et al. (2008). Common persistent pain conditions in developed and developing countries: gender and age differences and comorbidity with depression anxiety disorders. *The Journal of Pain* 9 (10): 883–891.

Wells, M., Aitchison, P., Harris, F. et al. (2017). Barriers and facilitators to smoking cessation in a cancer context: a qualitative study of patient, family and professional views. *BMC Cancer* 17: 348. https://doi.org/10.1186/s12885-017-3344-z.

Wilson, K.G., Eriksson, M.Y., D'Eon, J.L. et al. (2002). Major depression and insomnia in chronic pain. *The Clinical Journal of Pain* 18 (2): 77–83.

CHAPTER 6

Professional Behaviours and Culture

Ruth M. Strudwick and Amy Hancock

This chapter looks at behaviours exhibited by radiographers and how these influence their attitudes to patients and the care of the patient.

FORMATION OF ATTITUDES TOWARDS PATIENTS

The chapter will start by briefly considering how attitudes are formed, this will help us to understand how our attitudes can influence professional interactions with patients.

Attitude is often described as a feeling or opinion about something or someone, meaning our attitudes are towards or of a specific target or 'object', such as a person, place, material object, issue, or social group (Zanna and Rempel 1988; McCulloch et al. 2009; Cunningham and Luttrell 2015). To be able to form an attitude we have to undertake a process of evaluation of that object, this evaluation can be either conscious or unconscious and subsequently forms the basis of an opinion (Smith et al. 1956; Rokeach 1968). When we evaluate objects, we naturally do this along a scale of favour or disfavour, good or bad, like or dislike (Ajzen and Fishbein 2000). This is frequently described as 'liking' or having a favourable opinion of the object, conversely this can also be a dislike, or unfavourable opinion of the object (Allport 1935; Rokeach 1968; Ajzen and Fishbein 1975; Ajzen and Fishbein 2000).

Person-centred Care in Radiography: Skills for Providing Effective Patient Care, First Edition.
Ruth M. Strudwick, Jane M. Harvey-Lloyd, Jill Bleiker, Jane Gooch, Amy Hancock,
Emma Hyde, and Ann Newton-Hughes.
© 2024 John Wiley & Sons Ltd. Published 2024 by John Wiley & Sons Ltd.

When radiographers evaluate an 'object' as part of the process of attitude development and opinion formation, it is important for them to consider the 'object' is a patient who is attending for radiographic imaging or therapeutic treatment. Radiographers must also consider how liking a patient is not the opposite of disliking the patient and that it is also alright if we do not have or support the same beliefs or values or even 'like' the patient as a person as that does not necessarily mean we dislike them (Cacioppo et al. 1997). We must however not treat them any differently than we would any other patient.

JUDGEMENTAL ATTITUDES

As Chapter 5 highlighted, radiographers must manage and care for a spectrum of patients (from different backgrounds, cultures, belief systems, etc.) attending diagnostic imaging and radiotherapy departments. Clinical situations often highlight individual differences within all of us as human-beings and demonstrate the complexities around caring for patients from across society. Patients may engage in behaviours which portray how their attitudes, values, or beliefs contradict our own. This can lead to the formation of judgemental and unprofessional opinions and although attitude formation is a natural human process, it is important to reflect and consider our professional responsibility to the patient and not let our personal opinion affect the standard of service delivery and person-centred care.

The quotes below illustrate how judgemental attitudes can create a barrier to effective delivery of radiographic imaging or treatment and negatively impact upon person-centred compassionate patient care (Taylor 2020).

"Sometimes your own opinions can kind of influence it *[your behaviour]* because obviously in my case the radiographers just thought well it's free healthcare and like why would you complain about this treatment that you are getting for free and it's going to save your life and kind of just thought about it from a treatment point of view, like well you need to have treatment so, and then come for your treatment no matter what"

—Student therapeutic radiographer

"Blood in his stools, blood in his urine and other bits and pieces and probably at the time they (the radiographers) sort of said yes, that's normal. And then I think some people sort of look at him as a little bit of a, a bit needy, a bit of a moaner"

—Therapeutic Radiographer

As established in Chapter 2, it is important as radiographers for us to 'put aside' our own personal opinions and attitudes, and instead respect every patient as an individual. Perhaps we could argue that this is a professional obligation rather than a choice.

"Look at the Tomotherapy and head and neck patients you deal with, the real fringes of society. But we still, I think the way people *[the radiographers]* on Tomotherapy deal with it, with their patients, it's just, it's exemplary. It really is a, you know, a great example to everybody to have the support of the patients, even though we're probably aware that they are probably still drinking, still smoking, still got the habits that got them into this position"

—Therapeutic Radiographer

Reflective Exercise

Think about a patient you have engaged with that you perceived to be 'different' from you.
How did you interact with that patient?
Did this change because of the differences between you?
Are you happy with how you interacted with them?
What would you do differently if a similar situation occurred?

The next section illustrates some of the unprofessional behaviours which radiographers can engage in during their interactions with patients and we will consider how they can damage the therapeutic relationship between patients and radiographers. The chapter will conclude with how professional behaviours can be promoted.

REDUCTIONIST LANGUAGE

Patients from all walks of life attend for imaging or treatment for a wide range of reasons. Radiographers, in common with other health professionals (Murphy 2009) are sometimes guilty of labelling or categorising these patients based on information such as: age; gender; the examination or treatment for which they are attending; the nature of the injury or pathology for which they are being investigated or treated and the circumstances of the acquisition of the injury or illness and sometimes even the mode of transport by which they have travelled to the department (Reeves and Decker 2012).

Rather than seeing them as a person first with health-related anxieties and concerns, unfortunately such labelling (Strudwick 2016) may lead to stereotyping and stigmatisation. Goffman (1963) argues that these are related to unconscious expectations and norms, and although in some instances can provide useful 'shortcuts' for busy radiographers under pressure of time, may also lead to formation of negative or prejudicial attitudes.

The ethics of labelling and categorising patients are sensitive issues in current healthcare practice, particularly when the standard of care is under scrutiny (Francis 2013).

It is generally part of any culture or group to have 'types' of people and to categorise people into groups (Agar 1980; Atkinson & Housley 2003). When people meet for the first time, they tend to categorise one another. Once someone has been categorised, a decision is made about the type of person they are, then it appears to be easier to predict how they will behave and understand their actions. People use their expectations, images and impressions of people to label and categorise them (Madison 2005). Becker et al. (1961) in their seminal work about the culture in medicine use the term 'labelling' to describe how society defines different people.

Davis (1959) in his paper 'the cabdriver and his fare' says that cabdrivers develop a typology of cab users based on their appearance, demeanour and conversation. In healthcare this also applies, Holyoake (1999) describes how this same concept occurs in nursing.

The radiographer's role is both technical and caring but tends to be characterised by less time spent with the patients when compared to other professions (Murphy 2006). Therefore, the radiographer must make quick decisions about their patients. As the previous chapter (Chapter 5) discussed, the patient may be in pain or have experienced an accident, illness or be suffering side effects from their treatment. Categorising the patient into a typology can assist the radiographer in their decision making and planning for the radiographic examination or the required set-up and immobilisation procedure for their treatment (Murphy 2009; Reeves 2009). Categorisation is about workload, typifying patients helps radiographers to decide how the examination or treatment would go, how to address the patient and more crucially gives them some idea of how long the examination or treatment might take so that they could plan. In categorising the patient, based on previous experiences radiographers can make judgements about what to expect.

This practice can however contribute further to the loss of identify already experienced when they take on the patient role (Long et al. 2008). Patients are often labelled according to their medical condition, for example they could be called 'a total hip replacement' or 'a prostate'. This reductionist language, where patients can be referred to as body parts is endemic within radiography (Reeves and Decker 2012). The radiographer will scrutinise an X-ray examination request form or the patient's medical notes, which normally begin with the examination or treatment being requested, a body part. This reductionist language is also part of radiography education, so student radiographers are introduced to it early on in their training. Students become very quickly socialised into this way of referring to patients, and the culture where the patient is discussed in relation to the body part being imaged or treated, for example, the next one is a chest, or the next patient is a breast.

Various authors discuss how patients can be categorised as unpopular patients (Becker et al. 1961; Dodier and Camus 1998; Cudmore and Sondermeyer 2007). This in turn has a potential to affect the way in which they might be treated. For example, the unpopular or difficult patient may be labelled as such and not receive a high standard of care.

TASK FOCUSSED INTERACTIONS

Radiographers are very task-focussed during their interactions with their patients, they either need to produce a diagnostic image or carry out accurate treatment and this is the focus of their time with the patient. The radiographer is concerned about the product of the interaction, the radiographic image or successful treatment, and consequently it may appear that they do not care for the patient in the same way that other health care professionals care. Their relationship with the patient involves actions and is more concerned with the instrumental aspect of caring (Widmark-Peterson et al. 1998) and being careful and precise (Barnum 1998). Caring is a very difficult concept to define, as some may also see technical competency as being caring or compassionate towards the patient (Bolderston et al. 2010).

TRANSIENT RELATIONSHIPS

As has been mentioned previously, the radiographer spends a short period of time with their patients, and they need to build a rapport quickly (Bolderston et al. 2010). Time pressures and trying to stick to appointment times also mean that the radiographer has to be able to have good opening and closing skills with their patients to ensure that they are in and out of the examination or treatment room quickly. The relationship between the radiographer and the patient is very much a transient relationship; diagnostic radiographers might see a patient once and therapeutic radiographers see patients regularly for the duration of their treatment and may never meet them again.

STORYTELLING

During the day radiographers discuss their work with one another as they are doing it. They discuss their patients, request cards and patient's notes, their images and treatment plans, the patient's previous images, colleagues, the rota, and how to do things. This mainly occurs in the staff only areas of the department. Radiographers might discuss challenging patients with one another before they start an examination to obtain some advice and decide upon the best course of action. This discussion about work is used to gain reassurance and feedback from colleagues and is generally positive. Radiographers tend to learn whilst doing and use the experience and knowledge of others to support their practice. This fits with what Benner (2001) says about experience and expertise, she says that expertise develops when the clinician tests and refines propositions, hypotheses and expectations. Experience is a requisite for expertise and makes interpretation possible and that clinicians compare an experience with previous similar experiences. She concludes that experience is the refinement of preconceived notions and theory through encounters and situations. So, radiographers tap into the expertise of their colleagues by asking for advice or discussing a situation and those offering help and advice will often cite a previous, similar situation in their advice.

Storytelling about previous experiences is also commonplace amongst radiographers. These stories are often about other staff members or difficult situations and tend to occur during quiet periods within staff-only areas of the department. Radiographers might recall experiences or incidents that they had been involved in.

Sometimes storytelling sessions can become competitive, i.e. who can tell the 'best' story or to see who had the 'worst' experiences.

Brown (1998) in his book on organisational culture says that stories and storytelling are important parts of the life of an organisation. Allen (2004) suggests that a repertoire of stories and the ability to identify appropriate occasions for telling them are important requirements in becoming a competent member of an occupational group. Storytelling is about belonging. It can be used to justify actions to colleagues, storytelling can be used to explain why decisions were made.

Radiographers like to share their experiences with one another, and it appears to be part of the culture when in the staff room, viewing area or control room to tell stories and share experiences. Storytelling and listening to stories could be seen as an informal type of reflection on action.

However, storytelling might not always be positive. Discussions about patients could be negative and derogatory and this can be perpetuated.

FRONT AND BACKSTAGE

There are expected behaviours from staff in different areas of the imaging and radiotherapy departments. There is a definite delineation between areas where patients and radiographers interact with one another; such as the waiting area, corridors, X-ray rooms, treatment rooms which could be termed 'front stage', and areas where only staff were present, such as viewing areas, control rooms and the staff room which could be termed 'backstage'.

Behaviour in these areas is very different. Goffman (1963) likens our lives to a performance where we play a part and have some control over the impressions we portray to different people depending on the circumstances we find ourselves in. He says that individuals will seek to convey a certain impression of themselves to others. Individuals often 'play a part' and 'create an impression'. The 'front region' refers to the area where the performance is carried out, performers begin their 'act' when they reach the appropriate place and terminate the performance when they leave that place. The 'front' may include clothing, posture, behaviour, speech patterns, and facial expressions. A given social 'front' tends to become institutionalised in terms of the stereotyped expectations to which it gives rise, for example, a hospital, a library. When an actor takes on an established social role, he usually finds that his role is already defined. Goffman goes on to say that "the performer may be engaged in a profitable form of activity that is concealed from his audience and that is incompatible with the view of his activity which he hopes they will obtain" (p52). The 'back region' is the place where the performance is 'knowingly contradicted'. In the 'back regions' the performer can relax and drop his front. Different language is used 'front' and 'back' stage (Goffman 1963). It is in the 'back region' where radiographers use storytelling, dark humour, and joke together.

Murphy (2009) studied diagnostic radiographers working in a Magnetic Resonance Imaging (MRI) department and found similar results. He compared the department to a theatre using Goffman's work. He found that there were 'front regions' of the department where there was an audience – the patients, and 'back regions' where there was no audience. Murphy found a difference in language used and behaviour, he called their behaviour in the 'front regions' impression management where staff were conscious of the impression they gave to their 'audience'. It is similar to the way in which any person working with the public will behave, a professional 'front of stage' persona, and less professional and more relaxed 'backstage' behaviour. It is important to have this distinction so that staff have somewhere to relax and 'let off steam', where they do not have to keep up the act.

USE OF DARK HUMOUR

Like many other professions working in public services, radiographers use dark humour as part of their conversations about service users. This appears to be an acceptable part of their professional culture.

Dark humour is used as a coping strategy by radiographers to cope with the challenging and stressful things that they deal with at work, for example trauma, or the worst forms of cancer, the things that they find hard. They would normally cope with it by treating it a little bit more lightly and using humour. The use of humour gives the staff members a way of discussing something that has happened and bringing it out in the open in a non-threatening and less serious way.

Dean and Major (2008) suggest that dark humour serves to relieve tension, discussing the use of dark humour between staff on the Intensive Care Unit and how it is used to support peers and relieve the tension created by life and death situations. Dean and Gregory (2005) also found that humour was used to relieve tension within a palliative care setting. Higher stress levels amongst staff elicited greater use of humour.

Dark humour is only used in non-patient areas, and not within earshot of patients as it would be seen to be unprofessional and uncaring. Goleman (2004) suggests that dark humour is a way of hardening oneself to the emotional responses, handling empathy distress, joking about patients near death is part of the emotional shell, a way to deal with our own sensitivities. Radiographers use humour to deal with this emotion and harden themselves against involvement with their patients in order to protect themselves emotionally.

HOW DEPARTMENTAL CULTURES INFLUENCE PROFESSIONAL BEHAVIOURS

The cultures present in clinical imaging and therapeutic departments are as important as the individual radiographers who work within them for promoting professional behaviour. A culture is considered to be a shared set of basic assumptions, norms, values and/or repeated behaviours of a particular group (Dixon-Woods et al. 2014). Naturally radiographers (like any human being) will align themselves with the collective majority becoming socialised to 'the way things are done here' (Dixon-Woods et al. 2014). Subsequently, if the majority of radiographers within the department engage in professional behaviours then the culture becomes one which positively promotes professionalism. Conversely however, if the majority of radiographers engage in unprofessional behaviours, the culture becomes one which does not promote professionalism (Taylor 2020). This phenomenon is caused by subjective norms which are the perceived behavioural expectations of individuals or groups (Baron and Kenny 1986). Radiographers subsequently feel pressured to conform and behave in a way which they believe is expected of them by the collective in the department, in essence wanting to 'fit in' and be accepted (Taylor 2020).

Negative cultures can be changed through positive role modelling and by challenging colleagues who do not engage behaviours which do not represent the culture of the department.

ROLE MODELLING

Observing and learning from colleagues is a way radiographers can develop professional behaviours and continue to support a culture which promotes professionalism. Observing positive role models provides the benefits of personal motivation by seeing the positive impact on patients and allows for the development and attainment of wider skills, in essence a tool kit of how patients should be engaged with (Lockwood et al. 2002; Lankford et al. 2003). Shadowing those who are exemplars can inspire other radiographers to engage in similar behaviours. This can be achieved by illustrating an ideal, highlighting possible achievement they can strive for, and demonstrating the behaviours that should be employed with patients to be deemed as professional (Lockwood and Kunda 1997; Lockwood and Kunda 1999).

"I think that helps if everyone's kind of practising that and I learnt that watching in first year, watching all the radiographers"

—Student therapeutic radiographer

Reflexive Exercise

Think about someone you have worked with that you perceived to be pro-
fessional
What did you like about their behaviour?
How did the patient respond?
How could you emulate their behaviours/what could you learn from
them?

CHALLENGING BEHAVIOURS

Challenging the behaviours of others is never easy and could be even more
challenging whilst you are in training or working at a lower grade. It is however important that we all speak up, if you are unsure about what to do,
talk to a colleague or friend and ask for their advice. If a situation arises it
may be helpful for you to complete the reflexive exercise below which will
help you process what you witnessed and the key issues which the event
highlighted.

Reflexive Exercise

Think about a situation where you have observed unprofessional
behaviour
How did it make you feel?
How did the patient respond?
What did you learn from the situation about your own professional
behaviours?
Did you or could you have challenged that individual?

REFERENCES

Agar, M.H. (1980). *The Professional Stranger – An Informal Introduction to
Ethnography*. London: Academic Press.

Ajzen, I. and Fishbein, M. (1975). *Belief, Attitude, Intention, and Behaviour: An
Introduction to Theory and Research*. Addison-Wesley Publishing Company.

Ajzen, I. and Fishbein, M. (2000). Attitudes and the attitude–behaviour relation:
reasoned and automatic processes. *European Review of Social Psychology* 11
(1): 1–33.

Allen, D. (2004). Ethnomethodological insights into insider–outsider relationships in nursing ethnographies of healthcare settings. *Nursing Inquiry* 11 (1): 14–24.

Allport, G.W. (1935). Attitudes. In: *A Handbook of Social Psychology* (ed. C.A. Murchison), 798–844. Worchester, Massachusetts: Clark University Press.

Atkinson, P. and Housley, W. (2003). *Interactionism*. London: Sage.

Barnum, B.S. (1998). *Nursing Theory*. Philadelphia: Lippincott-Raven.

Baron, R.M. and Kenny, D.A. (1986). The moderator-mediator variable distinction in social psychological research: conceptual, strategic, and statistical considerations. *Journal of Personality and Social Psychology* 51: 1173–1182.

Becker, H., Geer, B., Hughes, E.C., and Strauss, A.L. (1961). *Boys in White – Student Culture in Medical School*. New Brunswick: Transaction Publishers.

Benner, P. (2001). *From Novice to Expert – Excellence and Power in Clinical Nursing Practice*. New Jersey: Prentice Hall.

Bolderston, A., Lewis, D., and Chai, M.J. (2010). The concept of caring: perceptions of radiation therapists. *Radiography* 16: 198–208.

Brown, A. (1998). *Organisational Culture*, 2e. Harlow: Prentice Hall.

Cacioppo, J.T., Gardener, W.L., and Berntson, G.G. (1997). Beyond bipolar conceptualizations and measures. The case of attitudes and evaluative space. *Personality and Social Psychology Review* 1: 3–25.

Cudmore, H. and Sondermeyer, J. (2007). Through the looking glass: being a critical ethnographer in a familiar nursing context. *Nurse Researcher* 14 (3): 25–35.

Cunningham, W.A. and Luttrell, A. (2015). Attitudes. In: *Introduction to Social Cognitive Neuroscience*, 235–239. Elsevier Inc.

Davis, F. (1959). The cabdriver and his fare: facets of a fleeting relationship. *The American Journal of Sociology* 65 (2): 158–165.

Dean, R.A. and Gregory, D.M. (2005). More than trivial: strategies for using humor in Palliative Care. *Cancer Nursing* 28 (4): 292–300.

Dean, R.A. and Major, J.E. (2008). From critical care to comfort care: the sustaining value of humour. *Journal of Clinical Nursing* 17 (8): 1088–1095.

Dixon-Woods, M., Baker, R., Charles, K. et al. (2014). Culture and behaviour in the English National Health Service: overview of lessons from a large multi-method study. *British Medical Journal Quality & Safety* 23: 106–115.

Dodier, N. and Camus, A. (1998). Openness and specialisation: dealing with patients in a hospital emergency service. *Sociology of Health and Illness* 20 (4): 413–444.

Francis, R. (2013). *Report of the Mid Staffordshire NHS Foundation Trust Public Inquiry*. London: The Stationery Office.

Goffman, E. (1963). *Stigma*. Engelwood Cliffs, NJ: Prentice Hall Inc.

Goleman, D. (2004). *Emotional Intelligence and Working with Emotional Intelligence – Omnibus*. New York: Bloomsbury.

Holyoake, D. (1999). Favourite patients: exploring labelling in inpatient culture. *Nursing Standard* 13 (16): 44–47.

Lankford, M.G., Zembower, T.R., Trick, W.E. et al. (2003). Influence of role models and hospital design on hand hygiene of healthcare workers. *Emerging Infectious Diseases* 9 (2): 217–223.

Lockwood, P. and Kunda, Z. (1997). Superstars and me: predicting the impact of role models on the self. *Journal of Personality and Social Psychology* 73: 91–103.

Lockwood, P. and Kunda, Z. (1999). Salience of best selves undermines inspiration by outstanding role models. *Journal of Personality and Social Psychology* 76: 214–228.

Lockwood, P., Jordan, C.H., and Kunda, Z. (2002). Motivation by positive or negative role models: regulatory focus determines who will best inspire us. *Journal of Personality and Social Psychology* 83 (4): 854–864.

Long, D., Hunter, C.L., and Van Der Geest, S. (2008). When the field is a ward or clinic: hospital ethnography. *Anthropology and Medicine* 15 (2): 71–78.

Madison, D.S. (2005). *Critical Ethnography: Method, Ethics and Performance*. London: Sage Publications.

McCulloch, K. and Albarracin, D. (2009). Attitude object. In: *Cambridge Dictionary of Psychology* (ed. D. Matsumoto). Cambridge: Cambridge University Press.

Murphy, F.J. (2006). The paradox of imaging technology: a review of the literature. *Radiography* 12: 169–174.

Murphy, F. (2009). Act, scene, agency: the drama of medical imaging. *Radiography* 15: 34e9.

Reeves, P.J. (2009). *Models of Care for Diagnostic Radiography and their Use in the Education of Undergraduate and Postgraduate Students*, 1999. Bangor: University of Wales.

Reeves, P.J. and Decker, S. (2012). Diagnostic radiography: a study in distancing. *Radiography* 18: 78e83.

Rokeach, M. (1968). *Beliefs, Attitudes and Values: A Theory of Organisation and Change*. San Francisco: Jossey-Bass, Inc. Publishers.

Smith, M.B., Bruner, J.S., and White, R.W. (1956). *Opinions and Personality*. New York: Wiley.

Strudwick, R.M. (2016). Labelling patients. *Radiography* 22 (1): 50–55.

Taylor, A. (2020). Defining compassion and compassionate behaviour in radiotherapy. Unpublished doctoral thesis. University of Exeter.

Widmark-Peterson, V., Von Esson, L., and Sjoden, P. (1998). Cancer patient and staff perceptions of caring and clinical care in free versus forced choice response formats. *Scandinavian Journal of Caring Science* 12: 238–245.

Zanna, M.P. and Rempel, J.K. (1988). Attitudes: a new look at an old concept. In: *The Social Psychology of Knowledge Cambridge* (ed. D. Bar-Tal and A.W.W. Kruglanski), 315–344. Cambridge University Press.

SECTION II

UNDERSTANDING THE SERVICE USER

CHAPTER 7

Diversity of Service Users

Jane M. Harvey-Lloyd, Jane Gooch, and Ruth M. Strudwick

What do we mean by the term 'service user'? You may think that it means patients and for many people using the department that is correct, but not everyone using the services of the department are *unwell*. Service users are anyone using the services of the department. *Who are they, who else does that include?* Think about who uses your department. There are no typical service users, no 'one size fits all' technique for providing care to people, so we need to think about who uses the service, what their needs might be, and how we can provide care for them whilst respecting their individuality and diversity, whatever it may be. In healthcare we demonstrate this by providing person-centred care and as mentioned earlier in the book, person-centred care is at the core of how we interact with service users. As health care professionals we have a duty of care to assess a person's needs on an individual basis, think about the care needed from their perspective and adapt the way we work. It is second nature to treat a child in a different way from an adult; you adjust your communication and behaviour to their level of understanding. Unfortunately, the needs of a service user are not always obvious. In some cases, there will be no information about the needs of the service user on an imaging request or referral form, so we need to understand this experience from their point of view. Communicating with service users in a way that is accessible to them and asking about their needs or preferences is the first step. We are creating an experience that will earn their trust and compliance to enable their treatment or imaging to be performed correctly. Above all we should preserve the dignity, respect, and individuality of the person.

Person-centred Care in Radiography: Skills for Providing Effective Patient Care, First Edition.
Ruth M. Strudwick, Jane M. Harvey-Lloyd, Jill Bleiker, Jane Gooch, Amy Hancock,
Emma Hyde, and Ann Newton-Hughes.
© 2024 John Wiley & Sons Ltd. Published 2024 by John Wiley & Sons Ltd.

Reflective Exercise

What do you think about when you hear the term 'Service users'? Would you be able to explain it?

What adjustments do you currently make to help support diversity amongst service users?

In these examples you may recognise service users that have been to your department, these are fictitious cases, based on real evidence.

PAEDIATRIC PATIENT

A six-year-old boy called Tom has been brought into the Emergency Department by ambulance and is accompanied by his schoolteacher. Tom was playing with a group of friends during his morning break, when he fell off a small low wall onto his elbow. He is in extreme pain and very distressed. He is calling for his mother. Tom has been very difficult to examine as he will not yet move his left arm and is holding it very close to his body. The triage nurse has given him some pain medication, telephoned his mum and is trying to make him a bit more comfortable. His mother is on her way.

On reading the request for his X-ray examination, the radiographer notes Tom's age and the circumstances in which he injured himself. She is also aware that at the moment, Tom's mother is not with him. After talking to the triage nurse, they decide that it would be best to wait until Tom's mother arrives before taking him into the X-ray room as she is only 20 minutes away from the hospital.

Once the radiographer is informed that Tom's mother has arrived, she gets the X-ray room ready before bringing Tom in. It is a busy day and there is a lot of noise, so the radiographer wants to bring Tom straight into the room instead of asking him to wait outside. The radiographer has been thinking about how best to communicate with Tom during the examination and she goes to fetch Tom and his mother from their cubicle. When she pulls back the curtains, the radiographer gives Tom a big smile and says a friendly hello. She then introduces herself using 'Hello, my name is.... (Granger 2013). The radiographer does not say her job title but explains in very simple terms to Tom what she is going to do and then asks him if he understands. He nods. Then the radiographer walks around with Tom and his mother into the X-ray room. Once in the room, the radiographer kneels down to Tom's height and undertakes the three required identification checks and gains consent for the X-ray examination to be undertaken from Tom's mother. The pain medication has helped Tom and although still reluctant to move his arm, he is much calmer. The radiographer then asks Tom if he has had an X-ray examination before. He has not. Next, she goes on to explain what is going to happen in a simple language that Tom will understand. Whilst she is doing this, she looks at Tom all the time and includes his mother. The radiographer asks Tom if he would like his mother to stay with him whilst he is having his X-ray examination, and he vigorously nods. Then she checks the pregnancy status of his mum before placing a lead coat on her. It is very heavy but brightly coloured with different animals on. His mum asks what animals he can see, whilst the radiographer moves the X-ray tube and positions Tom ready for his X-ray examination. The radiographer and Tom's mother talk to Tom all the way through the examination, reassuring him and explaining to him throughout. Once the images have been taken and checked, the radiographer goes back into the room and praises Tom. She gives him a choice of a sticker which he proudly sticks into this jumper. The radiographer walks back round to the cubicle with Tom and his mother and explains what will happen next. She gives Tom a big smile and says goodbye.

Let us examine this case study further:

- What do you think the radiographer did well in this situation?
- What type of language would you use when communicating with a six-year-old, so that they can fully understand your instructions?
- What aspects of positive body language did the radiographer use?
- If this child does not understand your instructions, how else could you explain to them what you need them to do?
- The radiographer took time with Tom and his mother to build rapport. What type of strategies could you use to build up a rapport with a child and their mother?
- What is the best way to check for understanding?

Engaging with and involving the carer of the child (in this case Tom's mother) is essential to the success of a paediatric X-ray examination. You should always ensure that you give the carer and child time, that you give clear instructions before, during and after the examination and that finally you clarify understanding. You may also need to consider other ways of imparting instructions to the child.

PATIENT WITH HEARING IMPAIRMENT

Mohamed attended the X-ray department for an X-ray examination of his right hip and pelvis, as he had been to see his General Practitioner (GP) with pain and discomfort in his right hip. The GP was querying osteoarthritis in Mohamed's right hip and had requested an X-ray examination.

Mohamed has had issues with his hearing for some time, but he has not sought any help with this. His family members are aware that he has a hearing impairment, and so they speak loudly when talking to him and are used to him saying 'sorry' or 'please can you say that again?'. He does not wear a hearing aid, but likes to lip read, he does not like to make a fuss about his hearing impairment.

When Mohamed arrives in the X-ray department it is quite noisy, and he has some trouble in hearing what the receptionist says to him, but he realises that he needs to sit and wait for his name to be called. Mohamed does not hear his name being called on two occasions, and so remains seated in the waiting area. After the radiographer has called his name twice with no response, he decides to go and speak to the receptionist who explains that she thinks that Mohamed may have a hearing impairment.

The radiographer decides to ask the male patients in the waiting room what their names are, until he finds Mohamed. Once he has identified Mohamed, he takes him to the changing cubicles to get changed for the X-ray examination. He explains what Mohamed needs to do to get ready and waits for him. Mohamed did not fully understand the instructions and appeared from the changing room with his gown on back to front and still wearing his trousers. Once this is rectified Mohamed is taken into the X-ray room and the radiographer checks his identity and gains consent for the X-ray examination. He speaks slowly and clearly, ensures that Mohamed can lip read and gives him the chance to ask any questions.

During the examination, the radiographer ensures that Mohamed can see his face and lips when he is giving him instructions and he focuses on him rather than trying to multitask. When he goes behind the screen, the radiographer ensures that Mohamed knows where he has gone.

At the end of the examination, the radiographer ensures that Mohamed knows how to obtain the results of the X-ray examination from his GP, and he knows where to get changed and how to exit the department.

Let us review this case study:

- There is some good practice and some areas that could be improved.
- Do GPs make any indication on request forms that a patient has a hearing impairment? Would this be useful?
- We cannot expect patients to tell us about their disabilities, some may be obvious, but others are hidden, and a hearing impairment is something that can be hidden unless the patient is wearing a hearing aid.
- Could the receptionist have made the radiographer aware that Mohamed had a hearing impairment before they called his name?
- Do we always rely on calling patient's names in a noisy waiting area? Is there something else we can do to alert patients?
- When we give a patient any instructions to do something, in this case getting changed, we should check understanding for all patients, but especially if we know that they may not have heard correctly.
- If we are aware that someone is lipreading, we need to position ourselves where the patient can see our face and lips clearly, we should not turn our face away from the patient and we definitely should not be performing other tasks such as moving the X-ray tube whilst speaking to the patient.
- Giving clear instructions before, during, and after the examination and checking understanding constitutes good practice for all patients

PATIENT WITH DEMENTIA

Frances is a 75-year-old female who has fallen at home where she lives alone. Her daughter, who lives nearby, found her on the kitchen floor that morning and called an ambulance as her mother could not get up and was complaining of pain in her hip. On arriving at the hospital, Frances has been examined by a doctor in the emergency department and he suspects she has broken her hip. He has requested pelvis and hip X-ray examinations to diagnose the cause of her pain.

The radiographers have the request form and go to collect Frances from her cubicle. They introduce themselves as Samiya and Rebecca, explain they are here to take her for an X-ray examination and want to check her details, but she is confused and agitated and does not know where she is. She tells them her name is Cissy but cannot remember her date of birth or address. Samiya checks the patient identification band that is on Frances' wrist to confirm her identity. At this point her daughter enters the cubicle and asks what is going on. The radiographers introduce themselves and explain why they are there. Frances' daughter confirms her mother's details and says that she prefers to be called Cissy. She tells the radiographers that her mother has Alzheimer's which is why she is confused; Rebecca thanks her and asks if she would like to accompany her mother to the X-ray room so that she is not on her own.

The radiographers take Cissy on the trolley and her daughter to the X-ray room. Once inside, Cissy becomes distressed; she does not like the dark room and grabs hold of Rebecca's hand. Samiya adjusts the lighting which seems to calm Cissy and asks her daughter to stay next to her whilst they position her. Rebecca speaks calmly and slowly whilst keeping eye contact with Cissy, smiling, and reassuring her she is safe, and that they are taking some pictures of her hip to see why it hurts. Cissy smiles back. Rebecca asks the daughter to come behind the control panel for the first exposure, but this unnerves Cissy. Rather than staying in the room, her daughter keeps chatting to her as the pelvis radiograph is taken, then returns to her side whilst they set up for the horizontal beam lateral hip projection. As the radiographers move the unaffected leg, they let her know what they are doing for this next image. The X-ray examination is completed; Rebecca says "well done, great pictures Cissy", as they take her back to the cubicle and explain to her and her daughter that the doctor will come and see them with the results. Cissy's daughter thanks them for their patience with her mum, saying she knows she can be difficult sometimes. The radiographers thank her for her help and let her know it made a difference her being there.

Let us examine this case study further:

- What difficulties might radiographers encounter when dealing with patients living with dementia?
- Why did the radiographers encourage Cissy's daughter to come into the X-ray for the examination? Did she need to be accompanied?
- Did the radiographers change the way they communicated with Cissy?

People living with dementia are part of every community, yet there is still a stigma surrounding this condition. The radiographers in this scenario gained the trust of their patient by demonstrating person-centred care and meeting her emotional and physical needs. They recognised that letting her daughter accompany her for the examination helped with the situation.

> **Reflection**
>
> How has this chapter made you think about your own behaviour in practice?
>
> Are there areas you feel unsure about?
>
> Many hospital trusts, universities, and schools have in-house courses and training to assist you in understanding the needs of our diverse service users.

REFERENCE

Granger K (2013). # Hello my name is. https://www.hellomynameis.org.uk/ (accessed 31 August 2022).

CHAPTER 8

The Role of Carers

Jane M. Harvey-Lloyd and Ruth M. Strudwick

WHAT IS A CARER?

A carer is anyone, child or adult who looks after a family member, partner or friend who needs help because of their illness, frailty, disability, or mental health problem and cannot cope without their support (NHS England 2022). The care given by this group of service users is unpaid. Many carers do not see themselves as carers and it takes them an average of two years to acknowledge their role as a carer (NHS England 2022).

It can be difficult for carers to see their caring role as separate from the relationship they have with the person for whom they care whether that relationship is as a parent, child, sibling, partner, or a friend.

Here are some recent statistics about unpaid carers in the United Kingdom (UK) (Carers UK 2021):

- One in eight adults in the UK are carers.
- Every day another 6000 people take on a caring responsibility – that equals over 2 million people each year.
- 58% of carers are women and 42% are men.
- 1.3 million people provide over 50 hours of care per week.
- Over 1 million people care for more than one person.
- As of 2020, Carers UK estimates there were around 13.6 million people caring through the Covid-19 pandemic.

Person-centred Care in Radiography: Skills for Providing Effective Patient Care, First Edition.
Ruth M. Strudwick, Jane M. Harvey-Lloyd, Jill Bleiker, Jane Gooch, Amy Hancock, Emma Hyde, and Ann Newton-Hughes.
© 2024 John Wiley & Sons Ltd. Published 2024 by John Wiley & Sons Ltd.

- People providing high levels of care are twice as likely to be permanently sick or disabled.
- 72% of carers responding to Carers UK's State of Caring 2018 Survey said they had suffered mental ill health as a result of caring.
- 61% said they had suffered physical ill health as a result of caring.
- Eight in ten people caring for loved ones say they have felt lonely or socially isolated.

Carers can also be paid workers and provide care for people in their own home or in a residential setting. There is a wide range of paid carers now in the UK, offering a variety of potential careers. Again, their primary role is to support people with all aspects of their day to day living which includes, personal care, social and physical activities, mobility, and mealtimes. This can include looking after; adults with learning disabilities, people with physical disabilities, people with mental health illnesses, those who have substance abuse issues, and the elderly. Carers can work in a variety of settings such as care homes, the community, and in people's own homes. Some carers sleep at the home of the person that they are caring for. It should be acknowledged that paid carers may also develop a close bond with the person in their care due to the nature of the role. Many individuals become very dependent on their carer.

It should be recognised that whether the carer is paid or unpaid, they are a vital asset to the NHS, but often do not receive the recognition and support they need. In 2013, NHS England held a Commitment to Carers engagement event. As a result of this event, a number of themes emerged which were found to be important to carers. These were as follows (NHS England & NHS Improving Quality 2014):

- Recognise and respect me as a carer.
- Ensure information is shared with me and other professionals.
- Signpost information for me and help link professionals together.
- Flexible care, available to suit me and the person I care for.
- Think about the whole family, including young carers and young adult carers.
- Recognise that I also may need help both in my caring role and in maintaining my own health and well-being.
- Respect, involve, and treat me as expert in care.
- Treat me with dignity and compassion.

THE RELATIONSHIP BETWEEN A CARER AND A SERVICE USER/PATIENT

As can be seen from the variety of people providing both paid and unpaid care, the relationship between a carer and a service user varies. Some carers are family members and therefore may have a close relationship with the service user, however this should never be assumed, and it is always best to check with the service user if they consent to the carer being present during their care pathway. It is also essential not to use the carer as a substitute for the service user, ensuring that primary contact and communication remains with the service user at all times.

One thing that should never be assumed is the relationship that exists. In our experience it is always best to ask the service user who they have with them and what their relationship is.

CARERS ACCOMPANYING SERVICE USERS TO THE IMAGING OR RADIOTHERAPY DEPARTMENT

Carers often accompany service users to hospital and medical appointments to provide support, help with transport, assist with moving and handling and provide communication support amongst other things.

Carers and service users may be happy for an accompanying carer to participate in the appointment, or they may wish for the carer not to be involved. The service user/patient should be able to express their wishes and choices and these need to be respected.

CONSENT

It is part of a radiographer's legal and ethical responsibility to ensure that consent is given by the service user before starting any treatment or investigation. This reflects the right that patients have over what happens to their own body and underpins person-centred care. For consent to be valid, it must be given voluntarily by an appropriately informed person who has the capacity to consent to the intended examination or treatment. Generally, this will be the service user or if under 18 years of age someone with parental responsibility. In other cases, it may well be someone who is authorised to give consent on behalf of someone else under a Lasting Power of Attorney (LPA), as a consultee or someone who is a court appointed deputy.

Therefore, in normal circumstances, the carer should not be giving consent on behalf of the service user but may well listen and give advice to the service user if needed. At the outset, that is why it is important to establish what the service user-carer relationship is. Ascertaining the capacity of the service user must always be a priority for the radiographer before commencing with any treatment or investigation. The service user should always give consent unless they lack capacity to do so, but the carer may be involved in communicating this consent. However, the service user may wish to go against the wishes of the carer, and the service user's voice must always be heard and prioritised. There are however times where this may be different, and the carer is the person that gives consent as stated above.

CONFIDENTIALITY AND SAFEGUARDING ISSUES

There may be occasions where a service user does not wish to share information about their condition or their treatment with their carer. We need to respect their wishes and ensure that we do not disclose anything confidential to the carer without the service user's permission. We would suggest that if you are unsure, you check with the service user before giving information to the carer.

There have been occasions where there are safeguarding issues which involve carers, for example they have been abusing the service user. An imaging examination or radiotherapy treatment session may provide the opportunity for the service user to be alone with the radiographer and be able to disclose something about the carer when they are not present. We need to be aware of this and listen to and observe our service users and their concerns.

INVOLVING AND VALUING CARERS

Carers can be an invaluable resource. We can use their skills and knowledge in assisting with our service users. Carers should not just be 'allowed' but should be welcomed into the hospital and that they have a right *but not a duty* to continue to care. It is a subtle argument but an important one and again this may help us to gain a deeper affinity for the 'carer's voice'.

We need to remember that carers are also service users and acknowledge their thoughts and feelings too.

CONCLUSIONS

Carers often accompany service users to hospital appointments. The definition of a carer is wide and varied, and carers can range from being family members to paid carers. It is important to establish what the relationship is between the service user and the carer and not to make assumptions. Always take the lead from the service user about how much they want their carer to be involved in their imaging examination or radiotherapy treatment.

Carers can be an important resource and source of information and we need to ensure that they are included if the service user consents to their involvement.

REFERENCES

Carers UK (2021). Facts and figures. https://www.carersuk.org/news-and-campaigns/press-releases/facts-and-figures (accessed 24 September 2021).

NHS England (2022). Who is considered a carer. https://www.england.nhs.uk/commissioning/comm-carers/carers/ (accessed 25 March 2022).

NHS England & NHS Improving Quality (2014). Commitment for carers: report of the findings and outcomes. Medical Directorate and Nursing Directorate. NHS England.

CHAPTER 9

A Conceptual Framework for Understanding Compassion in Radiography

Amy Hancock and Jill Bleiker

In Chapter 4 we aimed to untangle compassion from other concepts such as empathy and kindness in order to be clearer about their similarities and differences. In Chapter 5 we saw how pain and suffering consist of physical and psychological components, the importance of understanding the impact of these on patients and illustrated that depending on how patients experience pain we should modify how we care for them within our professional role.

Our attitudes to pain and suffering, as well as to those experiencing them are deeply rooted in our personal, professional and cultural values, and it is these which form the underpinning basis of the conceptual framework presented in this chapter. Values-based practice is discussed in greater depth in Chapter 12, there you will find exercises designed to reveal the things that matter to you, helping you to reflect upon your own values and consider their influence upon your practice and ability to give person-centred care.

As illustrated in Chapter 2, radiographers need to uphold the values to which we subscribe when we join the profession, espoused in the profession's Code of Conduct (Society and College of Radiographers 2013). This is easier when these coincide with our own personal values, not so easy if there is a mismatch.

Person-centred Care in Radiography: Skills for Providing Effective Patient Care, First Edition.
Ruth M. Strudwick, Jane M. Harvey-Lloyd, Jill Bleiker, Jane Gooch, Amy Hancock,
Emma Hyde, and Ann Newton-Hughes.
© 2024 John Wiley & Sons Ltd. Published 2024 by John Wiley & Sons Ltd.

Reflective Exercise

What do you consider to be your own personal values?

As these tend to reside in your unconscious mind, it is worth spending some time thinking about this and attempting to bring them into consciousness. You may at first think your personal values sit comfortably with those of the profession (Society and College of Radiographers 2018)/National Health Service (NHS) (Department of Health and Social Care 2021), but we are all human and each has a 'dark side' which can be difficult to acknowledge, but which may reveal itself when you are under pressure, stressed, or unhappy. Better to 'know yourself' now, than to discover the uncomfortable truth from feedback at your appraisal!

The conceptual framework which forms the basis for this chapter is shown in Figure 9.1. You can see that it consists of four components; we will explore each component separately so that you can understand how compassion is 'broken down' into very specific elements, each of which are essential if compassion is to be a part of person-centred care.

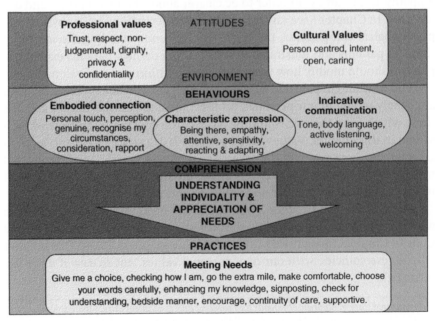

FIGURE 9.1   Conceptual framework for understanding compassion in radiography (Taylor 2020).

COMPONENT ONE: ATTITUDES

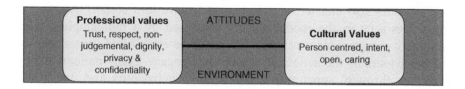

The first component of compassion is concerned with attitudes. You might also notice that these are all positive and reflect what patients want and need from their healthcare practitioner. Research shows that patients want to feel that their needs and wishes are respected, and that they are being cared for without judgement, whatever their behaviours or circumstances which have led to their needing your help (Taylor 2020). Patients need to feel safe, both physically and psychologically, and that they can trust that their radiographer will preserve as far as possible their dignity, privacy, and confidentiality. This means that radiographers' values must denote that they are person-centred, caring, open, and importantly, *hold an intention* to be compassionate.

Although these values are desirable characteristics of radiographers as human beings as well as professional practitioners, they also need to be supported by and reflected in the environment and ethos in which we practice, in other words our professional body, departmental culture and the wider organisation within which it operates.

Reflective Exercise

Consider the values of the NHS (Department of Health and Social Care 2021) and six Cs of compassion (Department of Health 2012)

If you have any experience of working within, or of being cared for by the NHS how far do you think the values of the organisation meet with your experiences?

Research suggests that many patients felt like they were on a production line, or that they were just one in a series of examinations or treatments to be performed that day (Taylor 2020; Bleiker 2020) and many reported feeling rushed and hurried through their procedure. How does that fit with the values promoted by the profession and by the NHS?

Our values underpin the attitudes we have to people and things and these in turn tend to dictate our subsequent behaviour. The professional and cultural values seen in the model must be possessed by radiographers if their corresponding practice is to be perceived as compassionate. Values and attitudes also dictate our *intention* to behave in a certain way, and if the values seen in the model are not possessed by a radiographer, then genuinely compassionate practice will never be established irrespective of the behaviours or the actions in which they engage. Some patients might even 'see through' apparently compassionate behaviours and detect the insincerity in the radiographer's behaviours or actions; ask yourself, how you might feel if you were a patient in that position?

In the next section we look at the specific behaviours which, if the intention is there, lead to perceptions of genuine compassion by patients from their radiographer.

COMPONENT TWO: BEHAVIOURS

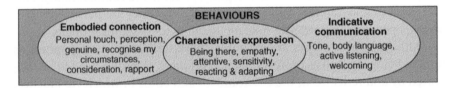

Embodied Connection, Characteristic Expression, and Indicative Communication are the core behaviours enabling radiographers to comprehend and interact with the patient as an individual. What do they mean? These are terms that we could usefully dissect in order to understand them better, beginning with embodied connection.

Embodied Connection provides radiographers with a tacit 'knowing' of the individual patient. This does not mean that we need to know their entire life story, just enough about them to be able to relate to what is happening and how they might be feeling. Some might say this is a little like empathy: an intuitive 'togetherness' which enables the radiographer to, if not instinctively then perhaps more readily respond with kindness and – if needed and wanted by their patient – compassion. You do not necessarily need to have had the same experience as your patient in order to make this connection; it is enough to have felt for yourself experiencing emotions such as fear, anxiety, worry, or sorrow – these are human experiences to which we can all relate at some level, unpleasant and difficult to acknowledge though they can be.

Characteristic Expression is a term for behaviours which are perceived as caring and which reflect how compassion is shown or perceived by a patient.

Research suggests these behaviours can range from the simple, such as smiling or greeting a patient, fetching a pillow or blanket to make them more comfortable, or more elaborate and time-consuming (Taylor 2020; Bleiker 2020). Have a look at the case study below for an example of how, although additional time was needed, a patient's safety and well-being was directly impacted by compassionate acts from radiographers and students.

Case Study: Compassionate Acts and their Impact on Patient Safety and Wellbeing

A patient attending for a barium study seemed understandably anxious and nervous, so the radiographers engaged in some light conversation aimed at putting them at ease as they waited to start the procedure. The conversation included questions such as "How was your journey here today?" and, having established that the patient was living in a care home, questions such as "Do you have a nice room?" slowly enabled the patient to feel safe and trusting enough to reveal some unhappiness about life at his care home. This raised concerns amongst the radiographers and led them to seek further advice before eventually the involvement of the adult safeguarding team was sought.

This is a good example of how what the students observing the interaction regarded as "just chatting" led to preservation of the patient's safety and wellbeing and how a compassionate 'putting the patient at their ease' can have far wider implications for our patients.

Indicative Communication is a term which refers to a dialogue and conversation that is understood by both radiographer and patient and facilitates acquisition of the knowledge and understanding that is essential in displaying compassion. Research suggests that the quality of the dialogue between radiographer and patient can range from minimal, such as checking the patient's identity and giving instructions, to wider and more personalised details (Bleiker 2020). These higher quality dialogues consist in part of personalised questions and attentive interest from the radiographer together with explanations about what to expect. These have been shown to calm and reassure patients and to help the procedure go more smoothly. As an aside, low quality dialogues also contribute to patient perceptions of radiographers as technicians or 'button-pushers' rather than expert professionals; which would you rather be seen as?

All three of these core behaviours; Embodied Connection, Characteristic Expression, and Indicative Communication hold equal importance, and each are essential parts of a compassionate display. Their undertaking symbolises to patients that the radiographer possesses those professional and cultural values which have been highlighted in this chapter and enables them to recognise and interpret them as compassionate care.

COMPONENT THREE: COMPREHENSION

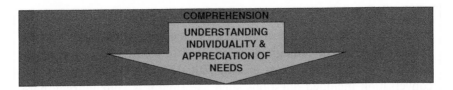

To comprehend a patient is to understand them as an individual with their own unique needs. Developing skills in reading and interpreting the verbal and non-verbal cues from patients is vital to this understanding and is key to a person-centred approach to their care (Taylor et al. 2021). Patients themselves do appreciate that although not easy, being able to recognise distress or discomfort is a component of compassion:

"It could be somebody ... they may not show the anxiety in the way that, you know ... you've got to be able to recognise the symptoms"

—Diagnostic radiography patient

Although research has yet to identify the precise skills that enable radiographers to be able to 'sense' a patient's emotional state, phrases like "picking up", and "reading body language" have been used; essential to these are close and careful observation of your patient from the moment you first see them. Students on placement started to notice patients' body language as seen in the example below:

"He was really showing that he needed someone to talk to"

—Student therapeutic radiographer

You may well find that skills in observing and interpreting patients' verbal and non-verbal communication cues (including body language) and your responses to them could develop with experience; radiographers contributing to the research that informs this book certainly thought so:

"your own arsenal [of responses to patients' verbal and non-verbal communication cues] also gets improved ... since you've experienced this kind of behaviour, this kind of approach. You also know how to choose, you know which one would be the right one to try, try one that doesn't work. Try the next one but as long as there are many options based on experience that will help you to a certain degree"

—Therapeutic Radiographer

Reflective Exercise

Ask a friend or colleague to communicate a feeling or emotion to you without using any spoken words. Practise interpreting their non-verbal cues such as facial expression, actions and gestures, and body language and then check in with them to see if you interpreted it correctly.

How did you get on? If you interpreted them correctly, what were the clues that gave away their feelings? If not, do not worry, it seems that we are primed, but not born to understand non-verbal communication cues and misinterpretation and miscommunication are common causes of unhappiness and dissatisfaction amongst patients – ask any departmental manager who is tasked with handling patient complaints. In the final section we explore the specific practices radiographers can undertake which lead to perceptions of a compassionate and caring encounter between patient and radiographer.

COMPONENT FOUR: PRACTICES

PRACTICES

Meeting Needs
Give me a choice, checking how I am, go the extra mile, make comfortable, choose your words carefully, enhancing my knowledge, signposting, check for understanding, bedside manner, encourage, continuity of care, supportive.

Meeting patients' needs, particularly the need to suffer as little physical and psychological or emotional suffering as possible is achieved ultimately by the engagement in practices by radiographers which are intended to give compassionate care to a patient. Compassion does not flow if a need is too well hidden by the patient, who may not wish to "make a fuss" or who's upbringing perhaps led them to believe that a public display of feelings and emotions is unacceptable behaviour. Compassion is also inhibited if signs given off by patients are not noticed by the radiographer, or worse, noticed but then ignored, perhaps in the rush to speed the patient through the department. The conceptual framework demonstrates just some of the things that radiographers can do that represent a display of compassion, but in this section, we use the reflective exercise so that you can start to develop your own personal arsenal of actions and behaviours, based on values of caring about your patient and respecting them and their dignity, as well as their privacy and meeting their needs whether visible or hidden.

Reflective Exercise

How would *you* give a patient choice, or 'go the extra mile' for them – do you have time for that in a busy department with a waiting room full of not-so-patient patients outside? Do they seem uncomfortable? In what way? Are you going to do anything about it or press on in the interests of a speedy examination/treatment?

How do you choose your words carefully? Imagine you have completed the examination/treatment and you cheerfully say to the patient "All done, everything's fine!" How might the patient interpret (or misinterpret) what you have said?

How does enhancing your knowledge help with communicating compassion? (For a clue, go back and look at the third component again)

How can you show that you are being encouraging, supportive? Would you use words or gestures? How would you do this without appearing patronising?

This conceptual model, and your understanding of it, illustrates first that compassionate person-centred care requires sensitivity to, and an understanding of, a need for psychological as well as physical safety and comfort – something we can all relate to (or empathise with). Further though, it is the ability of radiographers to identify these needs specific to the patient in their care and the undertaking of those behaviours aimed at alleviating their suffering which will lead to perceptions of a compassionate encounter. Importantly though, the behaviours and practices themselves are most likely to be exhibited when underpinned by the values and attitudes identified in this chapter and based on the understanding obtained by skilful interpretation of subtle cues from patients. Finally, it is the intention to be compassionate on which those practices are based which permits them to be perceived as compassion.

REFERENCES

Bleiker, J. (2020). An Inquiry into Compassion in Diagnostic Radiography. Unpublished doctoral thesis. University of Exeter.

Department of Health (2012). Compassion in practice; nursing, midwifery and care staff, our vision and strategy. https://www.england.nhs.uk/wp-content/uploads/2012/12/compassion-in-practice.pdf.

Department of Health and Social Care (2021). The NHS constitution for England. https://www.gov.uk/government/publications/the-nhs-constitution-for-england/the-nhs-constitution-for-england#nhs-values (accessed 20 Feberuary 2023).

Society and College of Radiographers (2013). Code of professional conduct.

Society and College of Radiographers (2018). Values-based practice in diagnostic and therapeutic radiography a training template. (ed. Strudwick, R. and The Association of Radiography Educators). In collaboration with *The College of Radiographers & The Collaborating Centre for Values-based Practice in Health and Social Care*.

Taylor, A. (2020). Defining Compassion and Compassionate Behaviour in Radiotherapy. Unpublished doctoral thesis. University of Exeter.

Taylor, A., Bleiker, J., and Hodgson, D. (2021). Compassionate communication: keeping patients at the heart of practice in an advancing radiographic workforce. *Radiography*. https://doi.org/10.1016/j.radi.2021.07.014.

CHAPTER 10

Interpersonal Communication Skills

Jane M. Harvey-Lloyd and Emma Hyde

INTRODUCTION

Radiography has often been thought of and referred to as a technocratic profession and, as such, many students are first attracted to the profession by the technology used to acquire imaging and deliver radiotherapy treatment. However, as imaging and treatment equipment continues to evolve and become more autonomous, there is increased focus on how radiographers' roles are changing to become more centred on the complexities of the individuals receiving care, who often present with co-morbidities and additional needs. Limited time to spend with individual patients combined with the increased demand for services (which often presents capacity issues), means that the need to be able to communicate effectively with individuals receiving care has never been more important.

Communication can be divided into two overarching modes; verbal and non-verbal. Non-verbal communication (NVC) covers aspects such as facial expressions, paralinguistics such as volume and tone of voice, body language, eye contact, listening skills, proxemics (e.g. physical space) and the use of touch. NVC is equally, if not more important than the verbal communication and can be used to develop rapport, demonstrate empathy and understanding, show acceptance, and reassure the patient and their carer(s). It is important to develop an awareness of your NVC to ensure that it positively reinforces the message being relayed. NVC can play five roles in the

Person-centred Care in Radiography: Skills for Providing Effective Patient Care, First Edition.
Ruth M. Strudwick, Jane M. Harvey-Lloyd, Jill Bleiker, Jane Gooch, Amy Hancock, Emma Hyde, and Ann Newton-Hughes.
© 2024 John Wiley & Sons Ltd. Published 2024 by John Wiley & Sons Ltd.

communication process; repetition (it can repeat and strengthen the verbal message), contradiction (this may indicate to the patient that you are not telling the truth or being insincere), substitution (at times it can substitute a verbal message, e.g. empathy), complementing (it may add to and strengthen the message e.g. a comforting or encouraging touch) and finally accenting (this can be the use of gestures to underline the importance of the message).

Regardless of previous experience, communicating with individuals receiving care and others is a skill that needs to be nurtured and developed. The premise of Neuro-Linguistic Programming (NLP) is that every interaction that takes place, has a positive intent. Meaning that as a radiographer, every time you communicate with another person, there is a reason for doing so and there is a purposeful, intended outcome to the interaction. How you communicate with others and the response you get when doing so indicates the success of that interaction. To provide person-centred care, radiographers need to ensure that the way in which they communicate is individually tailored and considers a range of influences that can affect how communication is received (Taylor et al. 2021).

The communication model used in NLP (Figure 10.1) can help us understand how we filter external events, and in particular information, according to our values and beliefs, our memories, experiences, attitudes, and language.

There are three main ways in which we filter information: deletion, distortion, and generalisation.

- Deletion is when detail is deleted from our awareness. This can explain why patient users often forget health professionals' instructions or explanations and why it is often necessary to repeat and reinforce information.
- Distortion is when we misinterpret or manipulate information. This often occurs in a stressful or unfamiliar environment and explains why although patients will follow our instructions, they will often do it in the wrong way, e.g. lay on the wrong side or change incorrectly for a procedure or treatment.
- Generalisation is when we take a small part of the information given and generalise it. This is not often witnessed by health professionals but often manifests in the non-completion of aftercare instructions when an individual decides that the instructions or information given was for everyone else but not them.

All these actions directly affect our internal representation of what we have been told or asked to do, which then drives our actions and behaviour

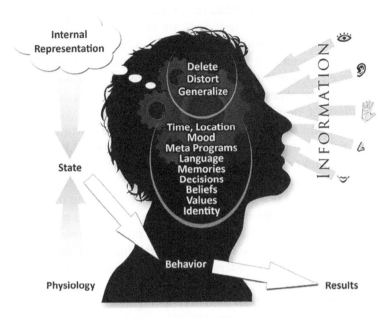

FIGURE 10.1   The NLP communication model (https://www.transformdestiny.com/nlp-guide/nlp-model-of-communication.asp).

accordingly. This goes some way to explain why sometimes the response you get from an individual you are caring for is not the one that you expected, even if you think the information you have been giving is clear.

Thus, having an awareness of the importance of influences such as values and beliefs will ultimately result in a more effective interaction. You may wish to revisit Chapter 2 which considers values and beliefs in detail and reflect on how this links with this chapter and your ability to communicate in practice.

Being an effective communicator takes time and practice and it is important to use all the information you have in advance of undertaking a diagnostic procedure or radiotherapy treatment. Taking time to consider individual circumstances and needs allows you as a radiographer to fully prepare for how you will communicate with an individual and meet their specific needs. It is easy to understand why lack of, or poor communication remains the major reason for complaints in the National Health Service (NHS) (Department of Health 2019), highlighting the importance of this aspect of the radiographer's role.

This chapter will introduce you to some fundamental principles you should adopt when communicating, using person-centred skills.

"The meaning of communication is the response you get"

- Purpose of communication related to the role of imaging/therapy professional.
- Importance and value of communication.
- Potential issues if communication does not meet needs of individual.

Before we move on to each aspect of the imaging examination or treatment, it is important to discuss the model of communication as this allows us to consider each part of the interaction with the patients and where it fits into this model (see Figure 10.2).

When undertaking communication during imaging/treatment, it usually begins with the radiographer as the 'sender'. In order to fully prepare yourself as the 'sender' and to correctly 'encode' the message you wish to send, the pre-examination/treatment considerations are essential. Spending time on this part of the procedure will ensure that you equip yourself with all the information you will need to ensure a positive interaction with the individual you are caring for and that the message you give is appropriate for the person in front of you. This includes how the information is delivered in terms of format and language. This interlinks with the principles of NLP (previously discussed).

Communication prior to and during the examination/treatment is the time when as a radiographer, you are most likely to receive feedback from

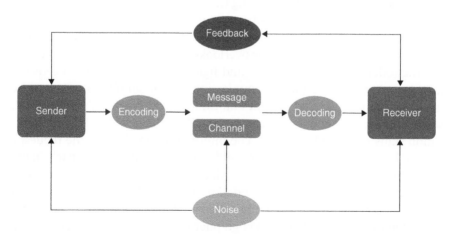

FIGURE 10.2   The communication process.   Source: Authored by: Freedom Learning Group. Provided by: Lumen Learning. License: CC BY: Attribution.

the patient. Sometimes, the receiver does not 'decode' the message as you expected, for example they may mishear your instructions or misunderstand them. Sometimes, the patient will ask for clarification and sometimes not. It is at this time that you need to learn to observe their non-verbal communication for cues that might tell you that there is an issue. When the message is interrupted or misunderstood, this is known as 'noise'. Can you think of any examples of noise that may contribute to this in an imaging and radiotherapy department?

If the patient has signalled that they have misunderstood you, you should at this point repeat the message a second time and follow this up with some questions to determine why the patient did not understand what you have said. At this point you may need to further explain something or change the way in which you are communicating with the patient. Reflecting on your practice at this point is essential to the success of your interaction.

The work by Harvey-Lloyd (2013) explored the use of Maslow's Hierarchy of Needs (Maslow 1954) in gaining the cooperation of paediatrics during imaging examinations (see Figure 10.3).

Harvey-Lloyd acknowledges that for there to be a successful outcome, the radiographer and child's carer(s) need to work together to motivate the child. This is easily transferable and can be applied to the communication process above with all service users. For the message to be decoded by the receiver, they need to be motivated to do so. At the bottom of the pyramid, the basic physiological needs must be met first, and this needs to happen with all individuals attending for either treatment or imaging. Pain management is an important factor and something that the radiographer can easily check with either the referrer or the patient prior to starting the procedure. There are other needs, some of which seem common sense but in a busy and pressurised environment, can often be overlooked, e.g. thirst, hunger, the need to use the toilet, noise, temperature, and lighting. Unless the basic needs are met, however effective the communication, it will simply not reach or be heard by the receiver and provides an unnecessary barrier. The next level, safety and security is one that can be heavily influenced by the communication skills of the radiographer. The information provided in the request / clinical history can be used to help build rapport with the patient early in the interaction, making them much more likely to decode the message that you are sending. This provides the foundation from which the radiographer can then start to give information to the patient and impart any instructions that may need to be followed. As a radiographer it is essential that you can use a wide range of ways to explain imaging/treatment procedures to patients and

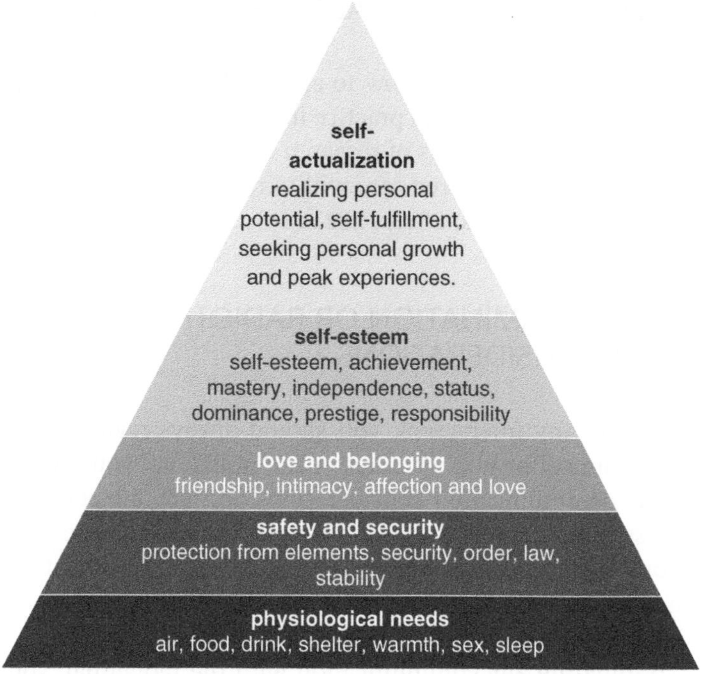

FIGURE 10.3 Maslow's hierarchy of needs (Tigeralee/Maslows hierarchy/CC BY-SA 3.0).

their carer(s) and to encourage them to ask questions. By doing this you are then obtaining feedback on whether the message has been received in the way in which it was intended. An understanding of the Hierarchy of Needs can therefore underpin your practice throughout the procedure.

Reflective Exercise

Think of a time when you were communicating with someone working in a service industry role such as a shop assistant, waiter, receptionist, etc., and you found it difficult to understand the communication they provided, or you received a response you were not expecting. How did that feel? What could they have done differently to aid your understanding of the information they provided or their instructions? How did your hierarchy of needs impact on this?

HOW DOES THIS APPLY TO RADIOGRAPHIC PRACTICE?

In this section we will consider how to apply NLP approaches to pre, during and post examination clinical practice in imaging and radiotherapy. This section draws upon the findings of research carried out in the UK by Hyde and Hardy about patient-centred care within radiography (Hyde and Hardy 2020; Hyde and Hardy 2021a, 2021b, 2021c).

PRE-IMAGING EXAMINATION OR RADIOTHERAPY TREATMENT CONSIDERATIONS

Before beginning any interaction, you should always review the request/referral form, clinical history, or notes of the individual you are caring for. This may flag communication considerations and any adaptation of communication style that is required, for example, the need to use visual cues, the need for a sign language interpreter, or the need for an interpreter to support individuals for whom English is not their first language, as well as any physical support needs.

Prior to initiating any communication with the individual, you should adopt an open posture, pay attention to your facial expression, and if appropriate use a warm smile. During this time, it is also important to use your observational skills to do a quick assessment of the individual to ascertain if they may require any additional assistance, such as support with mobilising. This is an essential part of building an initial positive relationship.

You should start any interaction with an individual with the use of 'Hello my name is . . . and I am the [insert role] who will be undertaking your [insert imaging examination/radiotherapy treatment]'. This is a simple but effective way to start any procedure which allows you to introduce yourself and your role before the examination or treatment begins. This phrase takes just a few seconds but is an incredibly powerful way to start to build a relationship, however short lived, with an individual. Using 'Hello my name is . . .' builds trust and confidence and helps to reduce the vulnerability that individuals may be feeling. At this point, it is also good practice to check how to address the individual you will be caring for and anyone that is with them, for example a family member, friend, or carer. This helps to further build trust and rapport.

Once introductions are made, you should take time to check that the individual and their family member, friend, or carer understand what is going to happen. You should ensure that you receive verbal confirmation that they understand the procedure and provide opportunities for them to ask questions. Active listening is key at this stage and gives you an opportunity to demonstrate your empathy for the individual. At this point it may also be useful to consider the use of silence. Research by O'Regan (2018) investigating the use of silence in radiography practice has provided evidence to support the use of compassionate silence to display concern for individuals. As part of the informed consent process the use of a compassionate silence can be useful to allow individuals time to think and ensure that there are opportunities to ask questions.

Once informed consent has been gained, then it is important to ensure any instructions which need to be followed are audible, or that there are alternative ways that instructions can be relayed. Consideration should be given to the use of hearing loops (where possible) and the use of visual cues. Ensuring instructions are understood is particularly important if an individual needs to change their clothing before their examination or treatment. Care should be taken to ensure that instructions about which items of clothing to remove, and what to put on, are clear, and that appropriate assistance to change has been offered. The clothing provided for individuals to change into should ensure that dignity is maintained. It has been identified by Hyde and Hardy that patients prefer hospital scrubs or tracksuits to hospital gowns, as they provide fuller coverage of the body (Hyde and Hardy 2021a, 2021b). However, if scrubs or tracksuits are not available then consideration should be given to providing dressing gowns instead. The safety and security of belongings should also be considered at this point, and lockers (or similar) readily available for clothing and valuables to be stored in during the procedure.

This is often a good time to also consider any specific support needs the individual may have. Allowing a family member or carer to be present during the examination or treatment whenever safely possible should be encouraged. A family member or carer is likely to know the individual well and therefore is best placed to provide the physical and emotional support throughout the procedure to achieve a successful outcome. Historically, many imaging and radiotherapy departments have discouraged family members and carers from entering the imaging or treatment room using safety issues as the rationale. However, there are many ways that safety can be ensured for family members and carers, such as wearing lead rubber aprons, asking them to stand behind the control panel during radiation exposure, or asking them to leave the room when the individual is comfortable and settled, and radiation is about to be administered. In Magnetic Resonance Imaging (MRI), safety measures would comprise the completion of a safety checklist, removing any possible projectiles and providing ear defenders. Although this may add a little extra time onto the procedure, it is time well used if it ensures the individual can tolerate the examination/treatment.

Finally, environmental factors such as lighting levels, warmth, music (if available), etc. should be discussed in advance with the individual receiving care, so that adjustments can be made to suit their preferences. This links directly with Maslow's Hierarchy of Needs which we have previously discussed, as ensuring an individual's basic physiological needs are met will underpin any successful form of communication and interaction (Maslow 1954).

DURING THE IMAGING EXAMINATION OR RADIOTHERAPY TREATMENT

Once the imaging examination or radiotherapy treatment begins, it is essential to ensure that good communication is maintained with the patient, and that the rapport established earlier in the interaction is nurtured. There should be continued opportunities for questions to be asked, and you should respond to these as fully as possible, and check understanding of your answers. Observation of the individual throughout the imaging examination or treatment is essential as it will also allow continuous reassessment of the individual, allowing you to pick up on any non-verbal cues which may tell you a different story than the verbal message you are receiving. This is particularly important when monitoring for pain or emotional distress. It also allows you to offer reassurance and comfort to the individual being imaged or receiving treatment knowing that you are with them throughout. This is particularly important during longer imaging examinations and radiotherapy treatment, as individuals may feel a sense of abandonment if regular interaction is not maintained. Simple interactions such as letting the individual know they are doing well, or how much longer the procedure will take, are particularly helpful.

It is also good practice to periodically check during the imaging examination or treatment that options continue to support the physical comfort of individuals, for example pain relief, warmth, comfort, lighting levels and music choice during the procedure. These interactions again link back to

Maslow's Hierarchy of Needs and ensure basic physiological needs are met (Maslow 1954). These can be key elements in ensuring a successful outcome to the procedure, which if not met, can result in the procedure needing to be stopped.

POST IMAGING EXAMINATION OR RADIOTHERAPY TREATMENT

When the imaging examination or radiotherapy treatment is finished, it is important to ensure the individual and/or family member or carer understand how they will get any results, and the next steps. Again, there should be the opportunity for questions, and the use of silence to allow thinking time. It is important to provide clear information to the individual and/or their carer about any potential side effects due to the examination or treatment, and any relevant aftercare advice, such as to drink plenty of water. You should check if the individual and/or their carer has any questions about potential side effects or the aftercare advice before they leave the department and ensure that these are answered as fully as possible.

You should also consider any safety aspects which may need to be highlighted to the individual and/or their carer, for example, relevant infection prevention and control measures, or radiation safety considerations. Radiation safety considerations are particularly important if the individual has had an injection of radioactive isotope as part of a nuclear medicine examination.

It may also be appropriate to consider signposting the individual and/or their carer to any sources of additional support, for example, Stop Smoking services, Drugs and Alcohol Support services, Alzheimer's Society, Macmillan Cancer Support, etc. A word of caution – this type of signposting should be done carefully and sensitively, taking a coaching approach, otherwise it can risk being mis-interpreted or seen as judgemental.

Assistance should be offered to support the individual to change back into their own clothing (if required), and consideration should be given to providing a wheelchair, calling the hospital portering service, notifying the ambulance transport service, etc., to help with the individual's journey home. You should also check whether the individual has any further specific needs which they require support with, before leaving the department, and that the individual and/or their carer knows the way out of the department before they leave. Consideration should also be given to signposting the individual and/or their carer to ways that they can provide feedback about their experiences, such as patient satisfaction surveys, comments boxes, etc.

Reflective Exercise

Thinking about each stage of an imaging examination or radiotherapy treatment, identify one or two areas of your interpersonal communication that you would like to improve. Think about how you could integrate these in your day-to-day clinical practice and create an action plan to help you do this.

SUMMARY

Communication is key to ensure a successful imaging examination or radiotherapy treatment, and provide reassurance, advice, and guidance to individuals in our care. It is reliant on not just the words we use, but also our non-verbal communication via posture, gestures, body language, eye contact, etc. which make up a significant part of our communication and interaction with individuals. Poor verbal and non-verbal communication can result in a sub-optimal experience for individuals and their carers and make them less likely to work with us to ensure a successful outcome. It is acknowledged that radiographers have often been viewed as a technically focussed profession, with the emphasis on producing a diagnostic image or delivering radiotherapy treatment. However, due to the number of people with complex needs now imaged or treated by radiographers, this balance needs to change to ensure we focus on the individual in our care rather than the equipment we are using. This chapter has introduced some techniques and models that that can be used such as Maslow's Hierarchy of Needs and NLP, these are ways that everyone working in radiography services can improve their communication to ensure a better experience for the individuals in our care and ensure a positive outcome to the interaction for all.

REFERENCES

Department of Health (2019). Written Complaints in the NHS 2019–20. https://digital.nhs.uk/data-and-information/publications/statistical/data-on-written-complaints-in-the-nhs/2019-20-quarter-2-ns (accessed 9 August 2022).

Harvey-Lloyd, J.M. (2013). Operating within the legal and ethical framework to gain co-operation when imaging paediatric patients. *Radiography* 19 (4): 285–289.

Hyde, E. and Hardy, M. (2020). Chapter 6 Patient centred care and considerations. In: *General Radiography: Principles and Practice* (ed. C. Hayre and W. Cox). London: CRC Press. https://www.routledge.com/General-Radiography-Principles-and-Practices/Hayre-Cox/p/book/9780367149871.

Hyde, E. and Hardy, M. (2021a). Delivering patient centred care (Part 1): Perceptions of service users and service deliverers. *Radiography* 27 (1): 8–13. https://doi.org/10.1016/j.radi.2020.04.015.

Hyde, E. and Hardy, M. (2021b). Delivering patient centred care (Part 2): A qualitative study of the perceptions of service users and deliverers. *Radiography* 27 (2): 322–331. https://doi.org/10.1016/j.radi.2020.09.008.

Hyde, E. and Hardy, M. (2021c). Delivering patient centred care (Part 3): Perceptions of student radiographers and radiography academics. *Radiography* 27 (3): 803–810. https://doi.org/10.1016/j.radi.2020.12.013.

Maslow, A.H. (1954). *Motivation and Personality*. New York: Harper and Row.

O'Regan, T. (2018). An account of silence in diagnostic radiography: a cultural quilt. EThOS.bl.uk/Home.do (accessed 22 March 2022).

Taylor, A., Bleiker, J., and Hodgson, D. (2021). Compassionate communication: keeping patients at the heart of practice in an advancing radiographic workforce. *Radiography* 27 (1): S43–S49. https://doi.org/10.1016/j.radi.2021.07.014.

CHAPTER 11

Is There More to Communicating with Patients than #Hellomynameis?

Jane Gooch

#hello my name is...

Too busy..sorry

We have all experienced less than satisfactory situations, whether it was in a restaurant or shop, where staff may have been rude or ignored you. Rather than recalling the nice clothes you bought or the delicious meal you ate, it is common to focus on the negative interactions and because of that, we choose to avoid returning there. Patients will often remember the interpersonal experiences they have with National Health Service (NHS) staff over the procedure or intervention (McDonald 2016). Patients have more confidence in health professionals that communicate effectively (Jones 2010). If you have an experience in healthcare where there was a problem with communication, or you did not feel listened to, to then avoid visiting your doctor's surgery or a hospital because of it, would be detrimental to your health and wellbeing (Figure 11.1).

Person-centred Care in Radiography: Skills for Providing Effective Patient Care, First Edition.
Ruth M. Strudwick, Jane M. Harvey-Lloyd, Jill Bleiker, Jane Gooch, Amy Hancock, Emma Hyde, and Ann Newton-Hughes.
© 2024 John Wiley & Sons Ltd. Published 2024 by John Wiley & Sons Ltd.

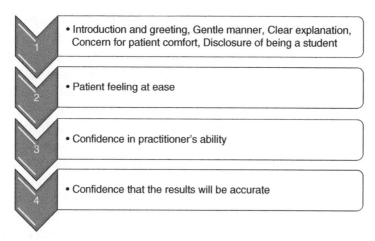

1 • Introduction and greeting, Gentle manner, Clear explanation, Concern for patient comfort, Disclosure of being a student

2 • Patient feeling at ease

3 • Confidence in practitioner's ability

4 • Confidence that the results will be accurate

FIGURE 11.1   Impact of effective communication on a patient undergoing an imaging examination (Pollard et al. 2019/With Permission of Elsevier).

In 2012 the NHS published a strategy which included the six Cs comprising: compassion, care, competence, courage, commitment, and communication (Department of Health/NHS Commissioning Board 2012). They are a set of standards for all health and social care staff to follow with communication being central to successful caring relationships and to effective team working. A year later, the Francis Report (Francis 2013) highlighted the lack of communication across the health-care system, which included interactions between health-care staff and patients. Poor communication can cause anxiety, distrust, and can lead to serious medical errors (Ali 2017).

When you meet someone for the first time it is natural to introduce yourself by saying hello and telling them your name. We experience this across the service industry, on the telephone, in letters, or in person, and as health-care professionals it is part of our role. It may seem hard to remember a time where health-care professionals did not wear a yellow badge on their uniform saying, "Hello my name is..." to identify their name and profession, yet the evolution of these name badges came from a patient who was frustrated at the lack of introductions by doctors and other healthcare staff treating her (Granger 2013). The irony of course is that the patient, Kate Granger, was also a practising medical doctor.

Communication is the key to a good workplace for those in our care and staff alike (NHS England 2015). As radiographers we follow the Health and Care Professions (HCPC) standards of proficiency which outline what service users should expect from their health-care professional, and standard of proficiency 8 focuses on effective communication (Health & Care Professions Council 2013). We are also required under The Ionising Radiation (Medical Exposure) Regulations (IR(ME)R) to communicate the benefits and risks associated with ionising radiation to patients (HM Government 2017).

In social situations we communicate with each other daily whether it is verbal or non-verbal, so why do we need to learn how to do it in healthcare, and how should we communicate with patients? Communication skills are mandatory in all medical schools in the United Kingdom (UK) and are part of the curriculum in nursing, midwifery, and allied health professional pre-registration degrees. As students prepare for clinical placements, they need to learn and develop these skills. Simulation-based learning gives students the opportunity to practise a wide range of situations that may occur whilst on placement. They can prepare themselves by being exposed to specific communication challenges such as grief, anger, anxiety, and diversity, which allows for discussion, debrief, and feedback with the outcome of effective communication. Once in clinical placement, students can develop their professional identity and observe the behaviours and attitudes of other healthcare professionals caring for patients.

A professional distance needs to be maintained whilst dealing with patients as we cannot interact with them in the same way we do our family and friends. Good communication is not always so easy and takes *more than "Hello my name is…"* it is the ability to connect with patients effectively that is core to our interactions with patients and is a key skill in radiography. There are many barriers and challenges unique to the profession, never more so than in diagnostic radiography and in some instances therapeutic radiography, where shorter, more focused communication exchanges with patients take place when compared with other healthcare professionals (Strudwick et al. 2011). Think about how long other healthcare professionals may spend with a patient and compare it to the duration of an X-ray examination or radiotherapy treatment. Within this time frame, radiographers are expected/need to explain a procedure to the patient and gain the patient's trust and cooperation to undertake the required task.

Therapeutic radiography staff may see their patients on consecutive treatment sessions, and most patients will spend longer with them than diagnostic radiographers. These patients will also be coping with a diagnosis of cancer and so radiographers will need to adapt their communication skills to provide both physical and emotional support for these patients, who may have undergone surgery, chemotherapy, radiotherapy, or a combination of all three (Kelly et al. 2021).

The first step in forming a connection with a patient is introducing yourself; failure to do this can occur when staff regard patients as a series of symptoms and tasks rather than as people with social and emotional needs which can leave patients feeling dehumanised. In radiography are your first thoughts when you pick up the request/referral form *'it's a femur on a trolley'*, or *'it's a prostate'*? Yes, they may be the clinical indications, but they should not define who the patient is. The person you are about to meet in the waiting room is someone you are about to provide care for, they could be one of your relatives: would you want them to be referred to as a procedure or a pathology, as discussed in Chapter 7. Patients need to believe that you are interested in them, and even when it is very busy, they need to know that they are not 'just another patient' (Taylor 2020).

After completing the identity check, we can ask the patient how they would like to be addressed; You might hear patients being called 'love', 'sweetheart', 'my dear', and although these are informal ways to address people, we should treat patients with respect and ask, 'what would you like me to call you?' Calling them by their preferred name even if it is a nickname, shows them you have a genuine interest in them as a person. They will feel reassured and more confident in your care. It can also demonstrate you are respectful of their diversity. Whilst in conversation with patients we may also learn facts that are relevant to their treatment or imaging such as a medical condition that has not been mentioned on the request form.

Patients want to know what is going to happen to them; what the procedure is, what it might find, will it take long, will it hurt? We are the gatekeepers of that knowledge and should anticipate any potential questions thrown at us. Some people will have had previous imaging or a therapeutic procedure and will know what will happen and their expectations may be high. Others will have anecdotal information from friends, family, or the internet, and this acquired knowledge can prove difficult as they will have preconceived ideas. It is our responsibility to correct their misunderstandings here are some common ones you may have heard in the department:

"Is that the one that is like being in a coffin?"
"Radiation is harmful, you're only allowed five X-rays in your life"
"Are they those lasers that shoot out of the wall and burn you?"

How many of you have heard similar statements to these genuine comments from patients? They highlight how one of the most powerful mechanisms through which communication can influence health outcomes is the impact it can have on our service users; it can help reassure them and reduce any anxiety they may be experiencing about their treatment, imaging, and radiation exposure.

Patients, like all of us, selectively process information and hear only what they want to and that is where communication can go wrong. It can break down for various reasons; is it the patient's situation? Are they worried about receiving the results of the imaging? Are they worried the radiotherapy will make them feel sick? Have they had a bad experience elsewhere in the hospital or is it just one of those days? We need to be mindful of what may be happening in their life as it could affect how they listen to you and how you communicate with them. Are there cultural or religious concerns that they feel unable to share, or are they embarrassed? Is it just information overload? As healthcare professionals that are used to the hospital environment, we forget how overwhelming it may feel to others. We can develop skills to read a person's body language and look for non-verbal signals that could identify a patient's concerns about their visit, this is discussed further in Chapter 7. They should guide you on how to help them through the procedure, whilst demonstrating empathy, compassion, and kindness.

Listening is as important as what we say – it is essential for "no decision about me without me" (Coulter and Collins 2011). Active listening will enable you to modify the information you give to the patient and decide if the patient has understood the instructions or the explanation you gave them. We have all seen patients put on gowns the wrong way round or lie face down on the table when we have asked them to lie on their back, because that is what they think they heard. If they have come to have their spine imaged or treated, they may presume that is what needs to be closest to the equipment. Positioning a person for a procedure will not always match the description in the textbook and we know from experience there is a need to adapt techniques or the treatment. In the same way, how we explain a procedure to someone cannot be verbatim terminology from a textbook. Explanations need to be adjusted for each patient, so they understand what you want them to do. There is nothing wrong with removing medical jargon from the conversation and simplifying the language we use to get the message across to the patient, e.g. 'I am going to take a picture of your chest and tummy' may be easier to understand than 'I'm going to image your thorax and abdomen' by some people; perhaps saying 'special X-ray dye to show up your organs' rather than 'an injection of contrast media' will help explain the purpose of it. Demonstrating the positioning required to the patient so that they can copy what they see is useful particularly where there are language barriers (Pollard et al. 2019). These suggestions may sound obvious, but sometimes 'the simpler the better' and by making reasonable adjustments to the way we communicate will consider the needs of people in our care. Repeating yourself, simplifying instructions or asking the patient repeat them back to you, allows you check that they have understood what you said and lets them ask questions if there is any doubt in their mind. Time constraints are often a barrier to communication. Taking the few minutes needed to reassure the patient is preferable to a rushed sentence which leaves the patient confused or concerned about what is happening to them. This includes how you end the procedure and the guidance you give the patient. This could be explaining what happens next, any post-procedure aftercare, and giving the patient the opportunity to ask questions if they want to. Your patient should leave satisfied that they have received personalised care.

REFLECTIONS

What communication challenges do we have as Diagnostic and Therapeutic radiographers?

By what means, other than talking to them, do you communicate with patients?

What adjustments do you make in your practice?

What do you need in the department to aid with person-centred communication? *Posters and visual aids, leaflets in a range of languages, translation service, National flags on name badges for multilingual staff*

How have your communication skills changed since you started clinical placements as a student?

How did you adjust your communication skills during the pandemic?

How could your place of education have prepared you for communicating with patients?

How have your communication skills changed with experience – what advice would you give yourself as a student?

How can you help prepare students for communicating with patients?

REFERENCES

Ali, M. (2017). Communication skills 1: benefits of effective communication for patients. *Nursing Times* 113 (12): 18–19.

Coulter, A. and Collins, A. (2011). *Making Shared Decision-Making a Reality. No Decision About Me, Without Me.* London: The King's Fund.

Department of Health/NHS Commissioning Board (2012). Compassion in practice nursing midwifery and care staff our vision and strategy, p. 13. https://www.england.nhs.uk/wp-content/uploads/2012/12/compassion-in-practice.pdf (accessed 24 April 2022).

Francis, R. (2013). *Report of the Mid Staffordshire NHS Foundation Trust Public Inquiry*, 1e. London: The Stationary Office London. https://assets.publishing.service.gov.uk/government/uploads/system/uploads/attachment_data/file/279118/0898_ii.pdf.

Granger, K. (2013). Hello my name is campaign. https://www.hellomynameis.org.uk/ (accessed 18 August 2020).

Health & Care Professions Council. (2013). Standards of proficiency: radiographers. https://www.hcpc-uk.org/resources/standards/standards-of-proficiency-radiographers/ (acceessed 20 Feberuary 2023).

HM Government (2017). *The Ionising Radiation (Medical Exposure) Regulations*. London: The Stationary Office.

Jones, J. (2010). Foreword. In: *Communication Skills for Adult Nurses* (ed. Kraszewski and A. McEwen), xi. Maidenhead: Open University Press.

Kelly, T., Thompson, J.D., Surjan, Y. et al. (2021). Lived experiences of first year radiation therapy students communicating with patients and radiation therapists – a qualitative review using interpretative phenomenological analysis. *Radiography* 28: 168–173.

McDonald, A. (2016). A long and winding road: improving communication with patients in the NHS. Bit.ly/MarieCurieLongWinding.

NHS England (2015). Compassion in practice strategy and the 6Cs values. https://www.england.nhs.uk/6cs/wp-content/uploads/sites/25/2015/03/cip-6cs.pdf/ (accessed 18 August 2020).

Pollard, N., Lincoln, M., Nisbet, G., and Penman, M. (2019). Patients perceptions of communication with diagnostic radiographers. *Radiography* 25: 333–338.

Strudwick, R., MacKay, S., Hicks, S., and Kelly, S. (2011). Is diagnostic radiography a caring profession? *Imaging & Therapy Practice* 4: 4–6.

Taylor, A. (2020). Defining compassion and compassionate behaviour in radiotherapy. Unpublished thesis. https://doi.org/10.7190/shu-thesis-00373.

CHAPTER 12

Values-Based Practice

Ruth M. Strudwick and Ann Newton-Hughes

INTRODUCTION

In Chapter 2, 'Exploration of your own values', we introduced values-based practice. We explained that values-based practice (VBP) is the consideration of the individual patient's values in making decisions about their care. We define a patient's values as the unique preferences, concerns and expectations that each patient brings to a practice encounter, and which must be integrated into any decisions about the care of the patient. VBP considers and highlights what matters and is important to the patient (Fulford et al. 2012).

In VBP we do not make assumptions about what the patient wants, and we also should not be reflecting our own values upon the patients we image or treat as radiographers. We need to be aware that what the patient actually wants may be quite different from what either the health care professional, or carer believes is in his or her best interests.

The 10-part process of VBP can be seen in Figure 12.1 below.

WHAT DOES VBP MEAN IN RADIOGRAPHY?

So, now that we know what VBP is, what does it mean in radiography?

Person-centred Care in Radiography: Skills for Providing Effective Patient Care, First Edition.
Ruth M. Strudwick, Jane M. Harvey-Lloyd, Jill Bleiker, Jane Gooch, Amy Hancock,
Emma Hyde, and Ann Newton-Hughes.
© 2024 John Wiley & Sons Ltd. Published 2024 by John Wiley & Sons Ltd.

The 10-Part Process of Values-based-Practice

Process is the 'engine' of values-based practice. Building on the premise of mutual respect, the process elements of values-based practice are what support its outputs in balanced decisions on individual cases within frameworks of shared values.

The process of values-based practice includes ten key elements covering four key **clinical skills**, two aspects of **professional relationships**, three close links with **evidence-based practice**, and a dissensual basis for **partnership** in decision making.

Clinical Skills

The four key clinical skills for values-based practice are awareness, reasoning, knowledge, and communication skills

1. **Awareness of values** includes awareness of the **diversity** of individual values, awareness of clinicians' **own values** as well as the values of others, and awareness of **positive values** (StAR values, i.e. strengths, aspirations and resources) as well as negative values (such as needs and difficulties)

2. **Reasoning about values** in values-based practice is aimed at **expanding our values horizons** rather than (directly) deciding what is right. Reasoning so directed may employ any of the established methods of ethical reasoning (such as principles reasoning, case-based reasoning (or casuistry), utilitarianism, deontology and virtue ethics)

3. **Knowledge of values** as derived from research and clinical experience has the important limitation that it can never 'trump' the actual values of a particular individual. That said, knowledge in values-based practice, as in any other area of medical knowledge, includes both tacit (or craft) knowledge and explicit knowledge; and it includes the skills for knowledge retrieval.

4. **Communication skills** include skills for **eliciting values** and skills of **conflict resolution.** In eliciting values, it is important to explore strengths (StAR values, i.e. Strengths, Aspirations and Resources) as well the standard ICE (Interests, Concerns and Expectations). So, in values-based practice ICE becomes **ICE-StAR**.

Professional Relationships

The two aspects of professional relationships important for values-based practice are person-values-centred practice and extended multidisciplinary teamwork

5. **Person-values-centred practice** is practice that focuses on the values of the patient while at the same time being aware of and reflecting the values of other people involved (clinicians, managers, family, carers, etc.): this is important in tackling two particular problems of person-centred care, problems of mutual understanding and problems of conflicting values

6. **Extended multidisciplinary teamwork** is teamwork that draws not only on the diversity of skills represented by different team members but also on the diversity of team values: this is important both in identifying the values in play in a given situation and in coming to balanced decisions about what to do.

FIGURE 12.1   Adapted from The Collaborating Centre for Values-Based-Practice in Health and Social Care (The Collaborating Centre for Values-Based-Practice in Health and Social Care, 2021).

Evidence-based Practice and Values-based Practice

The relationship between evidence-based practice and values-based practice is defined by three principles

7. **The two feet principle** is that all decisions whether overtly value-laden or not, are based on the two feet of values and evidence: clinically, this translates into the reminder to 'think facts, think values'

8. **The squeaky wheel principle** is that we tend to notice values only when (like the squeaky wheel) they cause trouble: clinically, this translates into the reminder to 'think values, think facts'

9. **The science-driven principle** is that advances in medical science and technology in opening up new choices (hence diversity of values) drive the need equally for values-based practice as for evidence-based practice: clinically, this translates into the reminder that above all in high-tech medicine it is vital to 'think both facts and values'

10. **Partnership**
    Partnership in decision-making, as the 10th element of the process of values-based practice, depends on both consensus and dissensus
    Consensus is when differences of values are resolved with one or another value being adopted (as in the adoption of a framework of shared values)
    Dissensus is where differences of values **remain in play** to be balanced sometimes one way and sometimes in other ways according to the particular circumstances presented by different situations.

FIGURE 12.1 (*Continued*)

All health care professionals have standards of proficiency. The Standards of Proficiency for Radiographers (HCPC 2013) (Statements 2, 5 and 8) clearly tell us that we must:

- Understand the need to respect and uphold the rights, dignity, values, and autonomy of service users including their role in the diagnostic and therapeutic process and in maintaining health and wellbeing (2.3).
- Understand the requirement to adapt practice to meet the needs of different groups and individuals (5.1).
- Understand the need to provide service users or people acting on their behalf with the information necessary to enable them to make informed decisions (8.5).

Radiographers can do this by giving the patient the opportunity to explain what is important to them; and by providing the patient with enough information so that they can make an informed choice. This is a critical aspect of truly person-centred care and VBP.

As we discussed in Chapter 6 with regard to reductionist language and labelling of patients, it can be easy to 'pigeonhole' patients and only consider the area of the body to be imaged or treated, e.g. "the next patient is a foot", or "there is a breast waiting". VBP reminds us that different people have different values, and these may be quite different from our own values or what we consider to be important. In addition, one person's values may vary from one appointment to another, depending on the situation and how they are feeling on that given day. Patients may value very different things from various practitioners. Therefore, it is important not to make assumptions about how a patient is feeling or what might be important to them. Each patient must be considered as an individual.

So, how can we embed VBP into our practice? The most obvious step is to get to know the patient and find out what is important to them. In addition, no decisions should be made about the patient without their involvement, 'No decision about me without me' (DH 2012).

For example, in diagnostic imaging the radiographer and patient can discuss how best to achieve the required images, and if any adaptation in technique is required. By explaining to the patient what is required, cooperation is much more likely with a good outcome for everyone involved. This might be allowing the patient to sit instead of stand or sit instead of lying down. Other examples might be negotiating a suitable time for an appointment that suits the patient, or consideration of the best location for the patient for them to get changed into a gown. These are all simple examples but give due consideration to what is important to the patient.

Back in Chapter 2 we asked you to complete the 'forced choice exercise'. It would be good to revisit this now and to think again about your own values and the impact that they have on you as a practitioner before you look at the next section which includes some scenarios from practice and some thoughts about the scenarios.

SCENARIOS

Mr Singh

Mr Singh attended the imaging department for a chest X-ray examination requested by his General Practitioner (GP) because of a persistent cough. Mr Singh was asked to undress in the X-ray room while the radiographer set up the equipment for the examination. Mr Singh removed his coat and shirt but was told he could leave his vest in place. The examination went smoothly and was soon complete. Mr Singh was asked to redress and leave the room while the radiographer tidied the room. Getting dressed took longer than the radiographer had anticipated as Mr Singh was taking a while putting his shirt back on. The radiographer stepped in to help and started to button up Mr Singh's shirt for him. Mr Singh objected strongly saying "he was not a baby" and turned his back on the radiographer insisting that he could dress himself. The radiographer apologised and waited patiently until Mr Singh had finished before ushering him from the room.

If we review this situation:
It is unclear why Mr Singh was asked to undress in the room – was this perceived as time saving by the radiographer or were they motivated by the impression that Mr Singh might need help in changing?
It is unclear whether Mr Singh was offered a choice in where he changed and whether he consented to change in the X-ray room?
Is it rude or unprofessional for the radiographer to set up equipment while Mr Singh is in the room or was the assumption by the radiographer that this would afford Mr Singh a degree of privacy and reduce the pressure of undressing that direct observation and waiting for Mr Singh might have created?
What was the radiographer's motivation in stepping in to help Mr Singh dress – was it to speed up his exit from the room and allow the room to be used again? Was it out of compassion for Mr Singh who appeared to be struggling with a routine task?
How did the radiographer communicate this with Mr Singh – was an offer of help made?
How did the situation make Mr Singh feel?
How did the situation make the radiographer feel?
Did getting Mr Singh changed in the room speed up the process or help Mr Singh?
Building rapport with a patient takes time – do we consider this when with our patients?

Mrs Jones

Mrs Jones came to the department for a chest X-ray examination. She had been referred as part of her clinical assessment for a hip replacement operation. Mrs Jones was shown to a changing cubicle where she was invited to undress down to the waist and wear a clean hospital gown. When Mrs Jones was invited into the X-ray room the radiographer noted that Mrs Jones was wearing a chain and crucifix around her neck. When the radiographer questioned Mrs Jones, she explained that for religious reasons she did not wish to remove the chain. On discussion with Mrs Jones the radiographer accommodated her wishes by clearing the chain from the area of interest and taping it to her cheek. The examination proceeded and both Mrs Jones and the radiographer were satisfied with the outcome.

If we review this situation:
Good communication allowed Mrs Jones to state her concerns and for the radiographer to find a solution to the difficulty.
This would have taken longer than conventional chest imaging as it would have taken the radiographer extra time for discussion with Mrs Jones and to find the resources necessary to help her.
Would it have taken less time if the radiographer had insisted that the chain be removed?
How might Mrs Jones feel after the examination?
How might the radiographer feel after the examination?
Are there other situations where patients are asked to remove religiously significant articles before examination?
Have we considered how these examinations might be adapted to allow religious observance?
For example, is it always necessary to remove a hijab for imaging of the cervical spine? Why do we ask for its removal? Is it to reduce artefacts? Is it to make positioning easier? Is it related to image quality?

Mrs Patel

Mrs Patel had been diagnosed with breast cancer and was referred for radiotherapy. The appointments clerk provided her with a list of dates and appointment times. When Mrs Patel attended for her first appointment, she asked if she could change her appointment times to midday. The radiographer listened to Mrs Patel and asked further questions to understand why. Mrs Patel explained that she had to drop off and pick up her daughter from school and she was concerned her appointments would make this challenging, especially due to her hitting rush-hour traffic. The radiographer reviewed Mrs Patels' appointment times and was able to accommodate her needs and schedule her in for the middle of the day whilst still ensuring that she would have her on-treatment reviews.

If we review this situation:
Good communication allowed Mrs Patel to state her concerns and for the radio-grapher to find a solution to the difficulty.
The radiographer listened to Mrs Patel's concerns and showed an interest in her values.
By listening to the patient, the radiographer identified further concerns and was able to suggest an alternative.
How satisfied might Mrs Patel have been if her request to change the appoint-ment time had been met?
How might this situation have been improved if an understanding of Mrs Patel's personal circumstances been obtained before for her first appointment?
How much do our appointment systems reflect the values of the patient?
Is it important to balance the patients' needs/requests with service delivery?

Mr Harris-Jones

Mr Harris-Jones was halfway through his radiotherapy treatment for head and neck cancer when he asked the radiographers if he could bring his hus-band into the treatment room so he could see what the machine looked like. He expressed that his husband was very anxious and becoming increasingly worried about what was happening to him, especially as he had to wear an immobilisation shell. He thought that if his husband could see what the treat-ment room and machine looked like, it may allay some of his fears and stop him imagining the worst. The radiographers looked at each other and simply replied no, it was not possible as the machine was busy.

If we review this situation:
The radiographers appeared to be rude/dismissive and did not consider Mr Harris-Jones' request,
The radiographers were not considering needs of patient/carer and the psycho-logical impact of the treatment on both of them.
How might this have made Mr Harris-Jones and his husband feel?
Why might the radiographers have responded in this way?
How might this situation have been more satisfactorily managed for all?

CONCLUSIONS

As can be seen the application of VBP is a process which brings together the values of the patient, the professional (radiographer) and evidence-based practice to form a partnership between the patient and the radiographer which allows an examination or treatment which satisfies the clinical requirements and reflects the needs (values) of all in the clinical context.

As radiographers we need to avoid allowing our own values to negatively impact upon the examinations or treatment we provide. Reflection on our practice can help us to understand how our values impact on our behaviour and the potential impact of these values on the experience of the patient.

REFERENCES

Department of Health (2012). Liberating the NHS: No decision about me without me. London: Department of Health.

Fulford, K.W.M., Peile, E., and Carroll, H. (2012). Essentials of Values-based Practice: Clinical Stories Linking Science with People. Cambridge: Cambridge University Press.

HCPC (2013). Standards of Proficiency for Radiographers. London: HCPC.

The Collaborating Centre for Values-Based-Practice in Health and Social Care (2021). *The 10-Part Process of Values-Based-Practice*. Oxford: St Catherine's College. https://valuesbasedpractice.org/more-about-vbp/resources-2/ (accessed 19 July 2021).

CHAPTER 13

Compassion in Practice

Amy Hancock and Jill Bleiker

In Chapter 4, we looked at what patients, radiographers and student radiographers think about what compassion means to them, and you may now have some ideas of your own as to this, and to the differences between similar concepts such as empathy, sympathy and care. In Chapter 9 we explored the theory developed from the research which has been undertaken into compassion in diagnostic and therapeutic radiography; in this chapter we apply this theory to radiographic practice.

One thing that everyone agrees is that for compassion to be considered part of patient care, or for an encounter between radiographer and patient to be said to be compassionate there are almost always observable behaviours and practices undertaken by radiographers that are designed to relieve a patient's suffering, whether that be mild discomfort, fear, worry, anxiety, or physical pain. We looked at some of these in Chapter 9 and here they are in Figure 13.1 below.

Reflective Exercise

Look back at the reflective exercises you did in Chapter 9 and refresh your memories of the ways you thought you might adopt some of the practices identified there. Then, think about how you would talk and interact with patients physically, verbally and emotionally whilst simultaneously undertaking the sometimes complex but mechanical and technical components of the task. Can you do both?

Person-centred Care in Radiography: Skills for Providing Effective Patient Care, First Edition.
Ruth M. Strudwick, Jane M. Harvey-Lloyd, Jill Bleiker, Jane Gooch, Amy Hancock,
Emma Hyde, and Ann Newton-Hughes.
© 2024 John Wiley & Sons Ltd. Published 2024 by John Wiley & Sons Ltd.

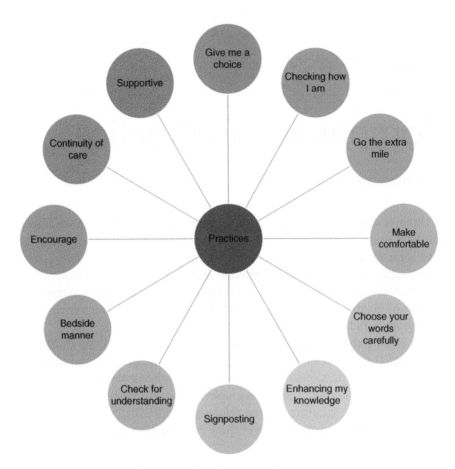

FIGURE 13.1   Compassionate practices (Taylor 2020).

On their own, and if repeated over time, these practices could be relatively easily achieved, a bit like undertaking uncomplicated imaging and radiotherapy delivery tasks until you feel quite confident. Then you are asked to image a patient for possible fractured elbow or treat a patient with a bone metastases; the problem is their arm is in a splint with the elbow fixed at 90° or they are lying on a trolley and cannot be moved, or they have difficulty hearing or understanding you, meaning that you will need to adapt your interpersonal and communication styles as well as adapting your radiographic/treatment technique – both at the same time – that is a lot of skills needed. So, it is important to get 'the basics' of compassionate communication established early in your practice so that they become second nature by the time the more difficult or challenging procedural aspects of radiography present themselves to you. That way you do not have to think about how you communicate compassionately with your patient and can focus on the task in hand – trust us; that will take up all your headspace!

For the rest of this chapter, we would like you to work through several reflexive exercises, which will help you reflect upon and develop your compassionate practices. You may not want to do them all at once, and that is okay, you can keep coming back to them when the time is right for you. Referring to Chapter 10 – Interpersonal Communication Skills can give you lots of ideas to start you off with these exercises.

COMPASSION PRACTICES: REFLECTIVE EXERCISES

Bedside Manner

We all nod in a knowledgeable way when we hear the term 'bedside manner', but what does it mean *in practice?* For this exercise construct a list of behaviours and actions that you think look like a good bedside manner.

First, think about what you would say to a patient (verbal communication) in terms of actual words you would use when talking to them. For example, would you say 'abdomen' or 'tummy', 'cervical spine' or 'neck' when referring to their body parts? Would you call them by their first name or something more formal?

Second, think about your non-verbal cues. Will you be looking at the patient or their details on the form or screen you are holding as you check their identity? Patients search their health care professional's faces for clues to help manage their emotions at this uncertain time. Of course, we all know the importance of smiling, but will you *remember* to smile, or might there be a small frown of concentration on your face that you are unaware of, as you contemplate how to image or treat this particular patient?

Third, body language. Open and facing the patient, or do you already have your back to them as you turn to enter and lead them into the X-ray or treatment room?

Check for Understanding

You have carefully explained the procedure to the patient, and they have not said very much. You ask them if they understand what is going to happen and they nod or say 'yes'. Why then, do they fail to co-operate or appear not to follow your instructions once imaging or treatment is underway? Patients are not unwise, but they are anxious, uncertain, and not in control of their situation and careful explanations are worth nothing if they are not heard and understood fully. So, other than asking them if they understand what you have said, how are you going to check that they *do actually understand* what you have told them? There is one really effective way of doing this, see if you can work out or find out what it is (*hint:* you will find the answer in the 'Enhancing my Knowledge' section of this chapter).

Signposting

You have just completed the procedure with a patient, when they start talking to you about a problem, for example they do not have enough pain medication to help them cope with their fractured hip or they have run out of anaesthetic mouthwash which they are using to help them to eat. Or they could be telling you they are struggling psychosocially, not sleeping and feeling low. At this point you may not be working in a role where you have completed any training to be able to give out medication or you may not feel equipped to counsel the patient through their struggles. So, what do you do? Do you just apologise and say you cannot help or is there something else you can do to illustrate that you understand their situation and are there to help? Are there people within your team, the department, hospital, or even the Trust to which you could refer patients to get the help they need?

Although the answer is in the name – signposting – and you may not have had to think too hard about what to do, it is important that we take a minute to think about the rationale and sentiment behind the practice of signposting.

It is essential that we make a distinction between accepting our limitations and appropriately referring the patient to someone else, as this is okay and safer for the patient. But what is not okay is not doing anything to help a patient because we have not got the time, as this can be perceived as 'passing the buck' and illustrates to the patient that we do not want to take responsibility for their care. The quote below is from a patient, here she is recalling what her doctor said to her when she explained she needed a physical examination.

"oh well if they think you need a physical examination they have got people at their end that can do physical examinations, you need to get them to sort one out for you at their end"

—Therapeutic radiography patient

How do you think this patient felt when nobody would accept responsibility for booking or undertaking the physical examination which was essential for her ongoing diagnosis/treatment? Hurt, frustrated, annoyed, and let down were just a few of the terms she used to describe her feelings.

As you will appreciate, we are all responsible as health professionals for a patient's physical, emotional, and psychosocial health, so we need to take responsibility for our actions and the needs of the patient. Appropriate and timely signposting depicts compassionate care as it illustrates to the patient that we understand their needs and the impact on them, that we want to help and that we are doing all we can to get them the help they need even if we cannot give it ourselves.

"If we can't look after them in that way, but we know somebody who can. So, it's just getting them the help"

—Therapeutic Radiographer

Think about some of the situations you have found yourself in where you have not felt appropriately equipped to help your patient, what did you do, how did you explain to the patient why you were referring them on and how did they respond?

Enhancing My Knowledge

We have started this section with examples from patients talking about their experiences during diagnostic and therapeutic radiography appointments.

"Nobody had told you how it was going to be"

—Therapeutic radiography patient

"hello, my name is ..., I'm here to give you an X-ray and you can find the results in a weeks' time if you phone up your doctor, but there was nothing like that so there was no information at that time or for the future. It was just very clinical, she was there to push buttons and off you go, but I didn't expect anything else."

—Diagnostic radiography patient

After reading these examples, can you understand why providing patients with information (i.e. enhancing their knowledge) is important? Think about the consequences for the patient of having or not having the information available to them, how would it have made them feel, how could it have affected their experience? Here is a clue:

"Yes, and having things explained, because I've always found if I know I'm reassured otherwise I'm worrying and thinking I'd rather know than not"

—Therapeutic radiography patient

Now consider all the different ways that you can provide patients with information. Think about when verbal communication involving telling the patient face to face might be more appropriate than providing them with an information sheet or vice versa, how would you decide which is the most appropriate? To help with this, think about the situation the patient is in, will they be able to retain the information you provide or have they already been overloaded during a stressful appointment. Is it something they need to know and act upon immediately or something for later in their pathway?

By being able to appreciate and understand the individual patient, their information needs and how those needs may differ in their current situation can illustrate that you are trying to enhance their knowledge to help improve their situation (or at least make it no worse). This is one way we can help patients holistically and portray a personalised, person-centred approach to their care.

Enhancing their knowledge also provides you with an opportunity to check their level of understanding; by asking them to repeat back what you have said to them. This does not need to be word for word, simply check if they are able to tell you the key points relating to the information that you have told them. If they are not able to, then now would be a good time to spend some time with the patient going through the information again to make sure they have grasped what you are saying. Investing this time now will help you both in the long run.

Checking How I Am

Patients are, for the most part are very keen to ensure that the imaging or treatment procedure goes well; after all, it is in their best interests to cooperate as best they can, despite feelings of discomfort, or pain. So quite often they will conceal these feelings from view. Reasons for hiding feelings and emotions can also include cultural norms, or stoicism. The evidence from these patients illustrates this:

"... that was two days after the hip replacement and it was still a... well I'm fairly bullish about things but it was still a relatively nervous time"

—Diagnostic radiography patient

"at the time I went in for that appointment, I was in the process . . . I'd been living with the pain for a while and going to see the consultant or going to see the radiographer ... was all part of steps that I had to take before the right diagnosis to be achieved and so I wasn't squirming, 'oh, that hurts,' or so I didn't really do anything that I would have thought evoked anybody to go, 'are you alright, dear?' kind of thing. I'm a little bit, kind of, deal with it and so I probably wouldn't have given any signals that I needed emotional support or reassurance or anything like that but I think I probably would have come over as a fairly confident person ... "

—Diagnostic radiography patient

So, how are you supposed to know how your patient is feeling if they do not tell you? Are they okay or are they struggling and need a particular act of compassion? Remember these can be 'little things' like fetching a pillow as in the case above – it does not have to be anything grander than that in many cases.

Think about how you are going to tell how your patient 'is'. Is it a simple case of asking them? (Answer: No; if you ask them if they are okay, the most likely response is "yes, fine thanks"). How else are you going to check how they are? If you need a clue, think about the non-verbal communication cues we have discussed in previous chapters. Is there a clue in their facial expression? Are they trying to communicate to you with their eyes? (You need to be looking at them and not the body part you are imaging or treating to even have a chance of figuring that one out). How are they holding themselves? Are they walking normally or is there something that suggests they are in discomfort or pain? Revisit the reflective exercise in Chapter 9 where you were asked to try and communicate specific emotions without using words and refresh your memory of the challenges of conducting that exercise.

Choose Your Words Carefully

We explored verbal communication cues in the bedside manner section, but what are other scenarios where careful choice of words is needed if misunderstandings are to be avoided? Have a think about what this patient had to say about their experiences:

"When I had, I think it was the first session, I think, or the second session of chemo, I was quite poorly. And for someone to say, what's wrong with you, it just made me so angry. Because you don't say to somebody what's wrong with you, it's the whole point and you can see it as well"

—Therapeutic radiography patient

You might think that it does not matter, no harm done, but the fact that this patient remembered this particular episode several years after it had taken place means that it had such significance for them that it stayed in their memory long after other details had been forgotten. This is called flashbulb memory (Brown and Kulik 1982) a snapshot in time which affects their perceptions of their experiences many years hence. The consequences of choosing your words carefully can be much longer-term than you might imagine. The words we use with our patients form the verbal component of the communication cues we use, for non-verbal cues see 'Reassurance' and 'Bedside Manner'.

Continuity of Care

What would you do if you had just collected a patient from the waiting room and were walking into the treatment/imaging room and you could hear your colleagues chatting about your favourite television show or the plans they were making for your team's Christmas party? What would you do if they asked you a question or tried to get your attention whilst you were with a patient? You may engage with your colleagues for only a couple of seconds – looking at them when they are talking, or you may answer their question. Is this the right thing to do?

What about if the question were work related, maybe about another patient or a radiographic task that requires your input, would you change whether you engage with them?

What do you think about this patient's experience, and what do you think can we learn from it?

"The nurse who was giving me the chemotherapy, somebody asked her behind her if she had children at home. And she carried on giving me the chemotherapy but talking to the person about her children and I said, actually, can I just stop you a minute, I said that's burning. And she looked round and said sorry, oh its fine and then carried on talking. Actually, it wasn't, it came back through and they had to stop and flush and she left the room crying, embarrassed because she had not given the time to the person she was dealing with, which was me, that was non-compassion"

—Therapeutic radiography patient

We all appreciate the pressures of the role and know it can sometimes be difficult as other jobs need doing and there is a queue of patients waiting, but it is important that we are consistent in the care that we deliver to patients. A key way to achieve this is to show patients that they have our full attention whilst they are in our care – this could be during their investigation/treatment or simply during an interaction on the corridor when they have stopped and asked you a question.

Another part of consistency is that we engage in these practices every day, which can be tough as some days you will have your own life pressures which can be weighing on your shoulders, or it may be that it is an extra hard shift as the department is short staffed.

"I think that's where it links in with patients as well it's got to be like a consistent thing, consistent sort of viewpoint that's ingrained into you. You can't just be compassionate on a good day, if you're having a good week at work, you've got to be compassionate on bad days as well which is probably the hardest part"

—Therapeutic radiography student

Reassurance

In the research we conducted for this book, we spoke with a lot of patients about their experiences of medical imaging or treatment (Taylor 2020; Bleiker 2020). Although many did not specifically mention feelings of anxiety, they did often use words like 'reassuring' and 'safe' which were interpreted to mean that in some way their radiographer had allayed their fears and anxieties:

"I felt safe in their hands"

—Diagnostic radiography patient

We may not have time to discover exactly what is going on in patients' minds, nor what is a particular concern for them, but having awareness that they may have specific, or more generalised feelings of worry can help us tailor our approach in a way that at least does not make things worse. Communication is central to this, but not merely the words we speak to our patients. As we have detailed in previous chapters, non-verbal and body language cues are just as important in helping patients feel safe in your hands.

Think (hard) about what non-verbal and body language communication cues can be used to reassure your patient. Imagine you are calling your patient in for imaging or treatment, right from the moment you first make eye contact with them. Work with a friend to act out how you are going to greet them, how you are going to speak to them, your posture, tone of voice, gestures, facial expression. You need to lighten a dark situation for your patient whilst striking a balance between appearing reassuring and friendly without being over-familiar or patronising – how are you going to do that? Take feedback from the person you are working with, and make sure that feedback is kind and constructive. You may feel a bit silly or embarrassed doing this, but these are vitally important skills to develop.

Extra Mile

Most of us are familiar with the term '*going the extra mile*', but what does that mean in practice? What sorts of things would you be doing for your patient for them to consider that you had gone the extra mile for them? You have a basic imaging or treatment task to complete. It is technically easy or difficult depending on your level of expertise, but that is really quite separate from the human being in your care. After all, you can position a dummy or mannequin in the classroom and master all the skills needed to perform the task, but the dummy just lies there … like a dummy. It does not feel hot or cold, uncomfortable, or in pain. It is not frightened or worried, fearful of the future, or regretful that it forgot to feed the cat before leaving the house this morning. It does not have family and friends who are concerned about it and what the outcome of this imaging or treatment might be. These are just a few of the human elements of interacting with patients that also need consideration and understanding if compassion is to feature in the care of your patient. So have a think about all those thoughts and feelings in your non-dummy patient's mind. They are cold; fetching a blanket would be an act of kindness, but there are none in the cupboard in the room and there is no-one around to ask if they can get one for you. It takes 10 minutes to go to the linen cupboard, find a blanket and give it to your patient. They could have been imaged or treated in that time, and you could be on to the next one (or at least another patient closer to your tea break). Do you fetch the blanket, or press on, justifying your choice by saying to yourself 'the less time they spend in the room, the sooner they will be warm?' From the patient's perspective, fetching the blanket is 'going the extra mile', not fetching it means lying there shivering while the imaging or treatment procedure is conducted and while waiting to find out if it is finished and they can leave. Something that seems like a minute or two to you can feel like a lot longer to a patient. Go the extra mile or get the job done as soon as possible? You choose, but remember it is not just about you …

Give Me a Choice

Thinking about the time you have spent with patients, have they asked you questions, wanted advice or your opinion?

Patients often look to us for help and guidance due to our professional training and knowledge, as quite often we know more about what is going to happen to them than they do. If we know better than the patient, then should we make decisions on the patients' behalf?

Absolutely NOT, this would not only oppose the principles of informed consent, but by not asking what the patient would prefer also contradicts the concept of 'no decision about me without me' (Anon 2011). Although you might think these principles only relate to the bigger issues like giving consent for treatment or for an investigation, these are an essential part of compassionate practice and the small things that we can do to engage patients in their care.

"You know it should really be up to the patient at the end what happens"

—Therapeutic radiography patient

"I want to be in the loop"

—Therapeutic radiography patient

In your daily practice, what can you do to make sure patients are engaged in their care and well informed about the decisions they are making?

MAKE PATIENTS COMFORTABLE

Although it may seem obvious, the quote below illustrates that if we can help to make patients comfortable, it may help them to maintain their position whilst undergoing imaging or treatment, subsequently helping them with physical comfort.

" . . . you don't want a fuss, so you quite often . . . yes, I have laid there in the most uncomfortable position sometimes, not wanting to say, 'have you got a pillow or two?"

—Diagnostic radiography patient

Similarly, helping patients to become emotionally comfortable (or you could say relaxed), when faced with the impact of having to attend for imaging or treatment (anxiety of visiting a hospital, fear of the unknown/what their imaging my show, will this treatment work, etc.), will help them to become psychologically comfortable and help support them to deal with the situation they are facing (which again may help them to maintain their position).

"I can remember because I remember feeling very comfortable so I know they must have been . . . I remember they were incredibly, very friendly."

—Diagnostic radiography patient

Both elements of comfort are extremely important and will help you to practice as a compassionate and person-centred radiographer.

Throughout this chapter we have tried to illustrate how these practices are often the 'small things', giving you examples of what these can be, providing you with the confidence to recognise patients' needs and be able to adapt in different situations with differing patients. What we have also highlighted is that it is sometimes easy to forget those small things when faced with the pressures of working in busy departments.

" . . . they shoved him on one of those trolleys and oh it was awful. They couldn't just put him somewhere where he would have been peaceful, they put him in the place where there were drunks"

—Therapeutic radiography patient talking about her father's experience

Take some time to think about some of the things you have or could do to help patients to feel more physically and psychologically comfortable. We are sure you will have already listed many of these as you have gone through the activities, but there may be more you have not thought about which are specific to this practice.

SUPPORTIVE

When we asked radiographers, student radiographers and patients/carers what compassion looks like they gave these answers:

"Sometimes that might just be like support"

—Student therapeutic radiographer

"Some kind of issue that they have needed your support"

—Therapeutic radiographer

"And I think that is, the support that I've been given is absolutely phenomenal, overwhelming in fact"

—Therapeutic radiography patient

You will have noticed that each group felt that support was an important component and something that could display compassion towards a patient. The difficulty is that support is quite a vague term and can encompass a broad spectrum of practices. Having a broad range of practices can however be a good thing, as it will allow you to adapt and tailor how to show support to a patient. Spend some time reading through this scenario and think about what you could do to help/could have done differently in this situation:

You are under pressure for time and your patient appears quiet and withdrawn as you image or treat them – you are grateful as it means you do not have to talk to them much and can get on with the task in hand. Much later your manager shares with you some patient feedback from a recent survey that indicates patients have felt that you were 'cold' or 'offhand' with them. This is upsetting as you feel that you are trying your best in challenging circumstances. Patients in our research mentioned things like 'a comforting arm' or 'reassurance of some sort'. How do you reconcile this with the pressures and demands you are under without becoming resentful or even bitter? How can YOU feel supported to give your patients the support they need?

MEETING NEEDS

As this chapter has demonstrated, it is important that you are aware of the patient in front of you and able to recognise what they are needing from you at a moment in time – established by employment of those behavioural skills discussed in Chapter 9. This may be nothing more than a straightforward explanation of the procedure you are about to undertake, or it may be something more complex like psychological or physical support. To help you to meet the needs of your patient you will need to use all the tools that you have in your arsenal, including your own skills, those of your colleagues and wider professional teams, as you must remember we do not work alone – we work as part of a team who care for patients. We must all accept however, that sometimes we are not able to fully meet a patient's needs, due to the complexities of individuals and situations. Research has however shown that for your behaviour to be perceived as compassionate by the patient, you do not have to necessarily meet their needs (Taylor 2020). This may sound counterintuitive, as a key part of being a healthcare professional is to help patients. What you must remember is that what we are considering here are practices that promote and display compassionate behaviour, rather than in addition to achieving a clinical goal (for example, a clear and well-defined radiographic image or a safely delivered fraction of radiotherapy). For patients, it is your underlying intent to be compassionate towards them that has made you engage in practices aimed to help meet their needs – these signify to the patient that you were trying to be compassionate.

As a final point, we need to refer to the conceptual framework provided in Chapter 9. As the last component of the framework, we must remember all that precedes the practical components required for compassionate display. The practices themselves are not compassionate unless underpinned by those attitudes and based on the understanding obtained by the behaviours that we looked at in Chapter 9. Take some time to revisit these and reflect on how your own attitude and subsequent behaviours have shaped how you practice and will these now change based on what you have learnt about yourself and how your behaviours are perceived.

REFERENCES

Anon (2011). *Equity and Excellence: Liberating the NHS*. Department of Health and Social Care. https://assets.publishing.service.gov.uk/

`government/uploads/system/uploads/attachment_data/file/`
`213823/dh_117794.pdf.`

Bleiker, J. (2020). An inquiry into compassion in diagnostic radiography. Unpublished doctoral thesis. University of Exeter.

Brown, R. and Kulik, J. (1982). Flashbulb memory. In: *Memory Observed* (ed. U. Neisser). W.H. Freeman.

Taylor, A. (2020). Defining compassion and compassionate behaviours in radiotherapy. Unpublished doctoral thesis. Sheffield Hallam University.

CHAPTER 14

Theoretical Models for Person-centred Care in Radiography

Emma Hyde

INTRODUCTION

In this chapter we will consider several theoretical models for person centred care (PCC) based on research carried out in diagnostic radiography by Hyde and Hardy (Hyde and Hardy 2020; Hyde and Hardy 2021a, 2021b, 2021c, 2021d; Hyde 2021a). Although the research was focused on diagnostic radiography, the findings are transferable to therapeutic radiography due to the similarities between the two professions, such as the use of equipment generating ionising radiation, the need for a balance between technical and caring skills, and the diversity of service users cared for by both professions. It should be noted that the research participants who identified themselves as patients or carers were known as 'service users' for the purposes of this project, hence the use of the term service users throughout this chapter. It is worth noting that although the research was carried out in the United Kingdom (UK), there do seem to be some similarities with radiography practices in countries such as South Africa, Australia, New Zealand, and Canada, due to the similar models for radiography education and similar scope of practice to the UK.

Hyde & Hardy's theoretical models were developed to represent the priorities of the five participant groups who took part in their research

Person-centred Care in Radiography: Skills for Providing Effective Patient Care, First Edition.
Ruth M. Strudwick, Jane M. Harvey-Lloyd, Jill Bleiker, Jane Gooch, Amy Hancock, Emma Hyde, and Ann Newton-Hughes.
© 2024 John Wiley & Sons Ltd. Published 2024 by John Wiley & Sons Ltd.

into PCC in diagnostic radiography: service users, clinical radiographers, radiography managers, radiography academics, and student radiographers (Hyde and Hardy 2020; Hyde and Hardy 2021a, 2021b, 2021c, 2021d; Hyde 2021a). The first model offered for consideration is a series of priority triangles. Five priority triangles are presented, one for each research participant group. Each priority triangle differs, depending on the aspect of PCC each participant group perceived as most important during an imaging examination or procedure. The second model is Hyde & Hardy's Model for Person Centred Care in Diagnostic Radiography. The priority triangles and model for PCC were developed from the data collected in Hyde and Hardy's research, and link directly to the themes and sub-themes identified during data analysis of responses to their online survey about PCC, which formed stage 1 of their research project (Table 14.1) (Hyde and Hardy 2021a, 2021b). The online survey used a series of paired attitudinal statements to explore participants' perceptions of PCC and provided a space for comments in a free text entry box. The attitudinal statements were developed from a document synthesis of key publications relating to PCC in the UK and tailored to reflect clinical practice in radiography.

PRIORITY TRIANGLES

The priority triangles were developed to represent the priorities of each different participant group, based on responses to an online survey. The priority triangles are based on Maslow's Hierarchy of Needs and place the fundamental needs of each participant group at the bottom of the triangle, with higher level needs occupying the higher levels of the triangle (Maslow 1943). The foundation for all of the priority triangles is the same – technical competence – as this was identified as fundamental to PCC by all five participant groups. However, after the foundation level, the priorities for each participant group differ significantly, illustrating how the perception of what is 'good' person centred care changes depending upon the role of the individual.

SERVICE USERS

In Hyde and Hardy's research, service user participants assumed that radiographers were technically competent to undertake their imaging (Figure 14.1), and hence this formed the foundation level of the service user priority triangle (Hyde and Hardy 2021a, 2021b). The next most important aspect of PCC

TABLE 14.1   Themes and sub-themes for PCC in diagnostic radiography. Adapted from Hyde and Hardy (2021b).

Control over environment	Use of technology	Comfort & care

Transportation
  Car parking – pay & display vs. pay on exit
  Support with extending stay if required
  Ambulance transport
  Public transport
	Professionalism
	  Confidence in skills
	  Technical competency
		Privacy & dignity
		  Gown sizes
		  Dressing gowns
		  Use of scrubs

Security
  of belongings
  of individual
	Explanation/Information giving
	  Use of appropriate language
	  Opportunity to ask questions
	  Information given about delays
	  Options provided if delay significant
		Communication
		  Opportunity to ask questions
		  Not feeling rushed

Waiting rooms
  Signposting
  Warmth
  Separate In/Outpatient Areas
  Quiet areas for patients with dementia
  Children's waiting areas
		Role of carer
		  Inclusion in examination
		  Support for patient

	Task focused
	  Efficiency
	  Waiting times
	  Focussed on equipment
	  Only considers own role in examination rather than whole patient journey
		Prioritisation based on need

Changing areas
  Curtained
  Door
  Straight into exam room
		Comfort & Care
		  Warmth
		  Positioning
		  Use of appropriate touch

Choice
  Chairs
  Gowns
  Blankets/pillows		

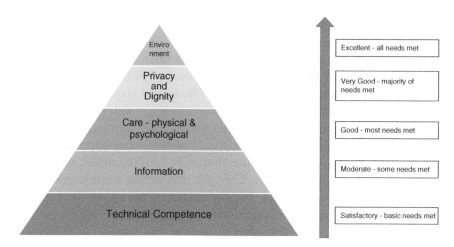

FIGURE 14.1 Service user participants priority triangle.

for service user participants was the expectation that radiographers would provide information about their examination or procedure, how to obtain the results, and details of any aftercare. As well as the delivery of information, time being available for questions (without being rushed) was noted as important. Service user participants placed importance on human interaction with the radiographer and on receiving physical and psychological care during their examination or procedure, such as a reassuring touch on the shoulder, and so this was their next priority in the triangle. Linked to this, and if possible, from a safety perspective, service user participants wanted to have a carer or family member with them throughout their examination or procedure to provide them with support.

The next priority for service user participants was the expectation that their privacy and dignity would be maintained throughout their examination or procedure. They highlighted the importance of considerations such as a choice of clothing styles and sizes, direct access to the examination room after changing (rather than returning to a waiting area), and provision of pads, pillows, and other items to help them maintain the position required. Linked to this, service user participants also expected to be offered blankets or duvets to help them keep warm, particularly during longer procedures.

If all their other needs were met, then service user participants started to notice the environmental factors such as the standard of the décor, information on noticeboards, provision of music, adjustment of lighting levels, etc. This element of PCC was therefore at the top of the service user participants' priority triangle.

CLINICAL RADIOGRAPHERS

Hyde & Hardy's research found that clinical radiographer participants saw technical competence as the essential foundation of PCC, which is the same as service user participants (Figure 14.2) (Hyde and Hardy 2021a, 2021b). However, above this foundation level, clinical radiographer participants saw their priorities for PCC differently from service user participants. Clinical radiographer participants saw efficiency as the next most important aspect of PCC, to manage the time pressures they were working under, and so this came next in the priority triangle. They felt that service users wanted to be seen as quickly as possible, and that any waiting times should be kept to a minimum. They also felt that appointment booking systems were organised to maximise throughput, and so keeping 'to time' was essential to ensure that the list did not run late.

Clinical radiographer participants understood the importance of communication and delivering information to service users about their imaging examination or procedure, and therefore this came next in their priority triangle. However, some participants indicated that they may avoid topics

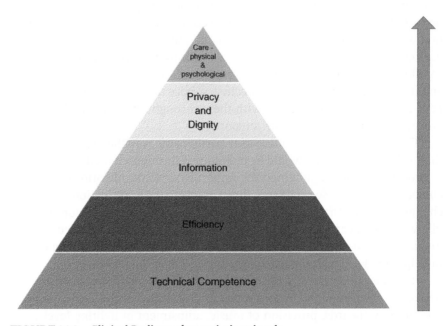

FIGURE 14.2   Clinical Radiographers priority triangle.

that could lead to questions that they did not perceive that they had time to answer. Clinical radiographer participants knew that maintaining service users' privacy and dignity was key to PCC but felt that they had limited time available to provide physical and psychological care, hence this element coming right at the top of the clinical radiographer's priority triangle. This finding reflected some of the challenges acknowledged by other researchers in radiography who have stressed the impact of time pressures, and the focus on technical aspects, on radiographer's abilities to provide high quality care (Bolderston et al. 2010; Strudwick et al. 2011; Bolderston 2016; Hayre et al. 2016; Bleiker et al. 2018; Strudwick et al. 2018; Hendry 2019; Taylor and Hodgson 2020; Strudwick and Hendry 2021).

RADIOGRAPHY MANAGERS

Radiography manager participants in Hyde and Hardy's research also expected radiographers to have technical competency at the foundation of their PCC practice (Figure 14.3) (Hyde and Hardy 2021a, 2021b). After this,

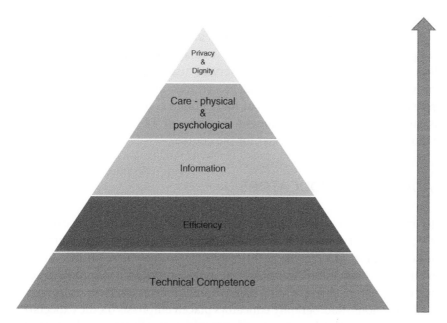

FIGURE 14.3 Radiography Managers priority triangle.

like clinical radiographer participants, their next priority for PCC was that radiographers worked efficiently and maximise throughput of service users. This is hardly surprising, as the way that health care services are set up in the UK at present, means that health care providers are paid for each 'activity' that they undertake (this is known as payment by results). This inevitably means that there is sustained focus on the number of service users that can be imaged or treated in any given time frame, to maximise income, rather than the focus being on the standard of PCC being delivered. The impact of these pressures is well discussed by Hayre et al. in their 2016 article about PCC in general radiography (Hayre et al. 2016). However, there was also some interesting discussion about the overall workload of clinical departments, and the time required to investigate complaints (Hyde and Hardy 2021b). Some radiography manager participants indicated that they felt that delivering good PCC was crucial to minimise the number of complaints received that required subsequent investigation, as this reduced overall departmental capacity, and therefore impacted on PCC (Hyde and Hardy 2021b).

Radiography manager participants' other priorities related to information, care, and privacy and dignity. They expected clinical radiographers to provide information to their service users about their imaging examination and provide opportunities for service users or their carers to ask questions. However, they also expected radiographers to interact with service users at a human level and provide comfort and care, to meet their physical and psychological needs. Radiography manager participants assumed that clinical radiographers maintained service user's privacy and dignity, in line with department policies and procedures, and as per Health & Care Professions Council and College of Radiographers Standards of Proficiency. As such, this was an afterthought in terms of PCC, as the radiography managers expected this to be par for the course.

RADIOGRAPHY EDUCATORS

The radiography educator participants in Hyde and Hardy's research also expected clinical radiographers to be technically competent as the foundation for PCC (Figure 14.4) (Hyde and Hardy 2021c). Their next priority for PCC for clinical radiographers was providing service users with information about their examination and providing opportunities for service users and/or carers to ask questions. Radiography educators placed emphasis on the expectation that clinical radiographers would interact with service users on a human level and provide high quality PCC which addressed service users' physical and

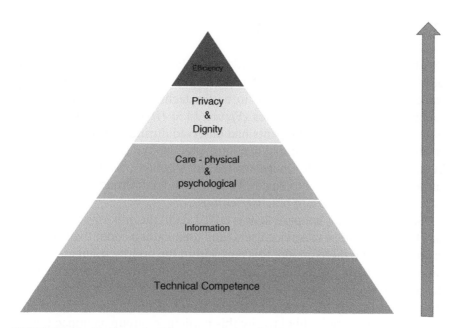

FIGURE 14.4   Radiography Educators priority triangle.

psychological needs. Radiography educator participants talked about the role of the carer in this, and some questioned why carers are often excluded from the examination room. Some educators stated that carers were usually the person that knew the service user best, and therefore could help to support them best.

Radiography educator participants expected clinical radiographers to always ensure privacy and dignity, as per their professional codes of conduct, and therefore this was high within their priority triangle. However, the pinnacle of their triangle was efficiency. Radiography educator participants acknowledged that there can be time pressures and a drive for efficiency within clinical departments but felt that this should not compromise or impact upon the way that radiographers cared for their service users. Some may argue that this is an idealistic view of clinical practice, and one that is unachievable with current clinical pressures. However, it is important to remember that although it may be your tenth chest X-ray examination or the planning of Computed Tomography (CT) scan of the day, to the service user the results of their examination could be life-changing for both the individual and their families. The radiography educators were very mindful of this, and the impact that PCC approaches could have on service users' experiences.

STUDENT RADIOGRAPHERS

The final participant group in Hyde and Hardy's research was student radiographers. Student radiographer participants were very clear that they expected the foundation for PCC to be the technical competency of both qualified staff and of themselves (Figure 14.5) (Hyde and Hardy 2021c). Student radiographer participants had observed during their clinical placements that efficiency is essential in clinical practice and talked about already feeling under pressure to image service users quickly. They therefore put this as their next priority to ensure PCC, which demonstrates the emphasis placed on efficiency within practice settings.

Student radiographer participants talked about the importance of providing clear information to service users (and their carers) about their imaging examination and therefore put this next within the priority triangle. Student radiographer participants also talked about how they strived to provide physical and psychological care wherever possible and maintain service user's privacy and dignity. However, again the issues of time pressures and efficiency on PCC were highlighted by this participant group as impacting on both aspects of PCC.

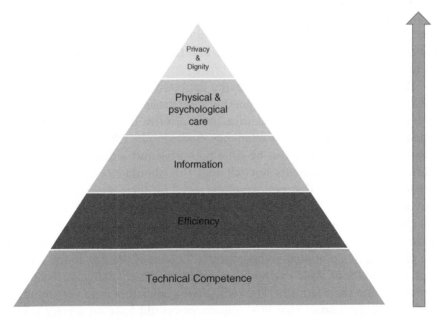

FIGURE 14.5   Student Radiographers priority triangle.

Interestingly, student radiographer participants' responses in the survey were the most closely aligned with the service user participants, providing a useful insight into PCC behaviours. Student radiographer participants also observed that qualified radiographers did not always provide the level of care that they expected to service users. As relative newcomers to the profession, student radiographers can perhaps provide a more independent view on PCC behaviours and approaches, which longer serving members of staff may not be able to due to the impact of time pressures and becoming part of the culture.

HYDE AND HARDY'S MODEL FOR PCC

The development of the priority triangles was a key part of the stage 1 data analysis during Hyde and Hardy's research project (Hyde and Hardy 2021a, 2021b, 2021c). After data collection and analysis of the focus groups and semi-structured interviews used in the second stage of their research, Hyde and Hardy refined their three themes for PCC in diagnostic radiography, and updated the titles of two of the three themes as follows:

1. Use of Technology – became Event Interaction - this more accurately reflected the sub-themes found such as task-focused, professionalism, information giving.
2. Comfort and Care – became Perception of Care – this more accurately reflected how participants perceived the care being given, and included sub-themes such as communication, inclusion of carers, choice of clothing.
3. Control over Environment – stayed the same and reflected issues such as transport, signage, security, waiting rooms, changing rooms.

This refinement led to the development of Hyde and Hardy's Model for PCC in diagnostic radiography (Figure 14.6) (Hyde and Hardy 2021b).

Hyde and Hardy's Model has been published in several peer-reviewed scientific journals and presented at several national and international radiography conferences (Hyde and Hardy 2021b; Hyde and Hardy 2021d). In addition, Hyde and Hardy have developed a Massive Open Online Course, or MOOC, which is an educational resource that can be used to increase awareness of PCC approaches (Hyde 2021b). Within the MOOC are several audit tools that could be used to measure PCC. The first audit tool is a self-audit which is an ideal Continuing Professional Development (CPD) activity that

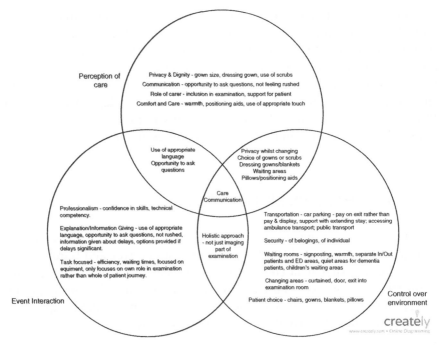

FIGURE 14.6   Hyde and Hardy's model for person centred care in diagnostic radiography (Hyde and Hardy 2021b/With permission of Elsevier).

could be used to demonstrate evidence of engagement in CPD. The second audit tool is for organisations to use to measure their level of PCC. This has been designed for use by radiography managers, clinical governance, or quality leads within departments, to measure the levels of PCC being provided, and support the case for improvement projects as required. It is hoped that this audit tool will support successful bids for funding for quality improvement projects which increase the levels of PCC being delivered to service users. Both of these audit tools are included in the Appendices of this book (Appendix A and B).

CONCLUSION

The theoretical models for patient centred care, MOOC and audit tools offered by Hyde & Hardy provide support for development of person-centred approaches, and a way to measure organisational responses to PCC. The MOOC and audit tools are available free of charge and could be used to drive quality improvement initiatives to support person-centred approaches, and for continuing professional development activity by individuals working in imaging or radiotherapy. The MOOC and audit tools could also be used to support staff development conversations and encourage a culture of person-centredness.

REFERENCES

Bleiker, J., Knapp, K.M., Morgan-Trimmer, S., and Hopkins, S.J. (2018). "It's what's behind the mask": psychological diversity in compassionate patient care. *Radiography* 24 (S1): S28–S32.

Bolderston, A. (2016). Patient experience in medical imaging and radiation therapy. *Journal of Medical Imaging and Radiation Sciences* 47: 356–361. https://doi.org/10.1016/j.jmir.2016.09.002.

Bolderston, A., Lewis, D., and Chai, M. (2010). The concept of caring: perception of radiation therapists. *Radiography* 16: 198–208.

Hayre, C.M., Blackman, S., and Eyden, A. (2016). Do general radiographic examinations resemble a person centred environment? *Radiography* 22: e245–e251. https://doi.org/10.1016/j.radi.2016.07.001.

Hendry, J. (2019). Promoting compassionate care in radiography: what might be suitable pedagogy? A discussion paper. *Radiography* 25 (3): 269–273. https://doi.org/10.1016/j.radi.2019.01.005.

Hyde, E. (2021a). Maureen's story: an insider's perspective on patient centred care. *RAD Magazine* 47 (552): 25–26.

Hyde, E (2021b) Patient Centred care in diagnostic radiography: an educational toolkit. Available at: www.derby.ac.uk/short-courses-cpd/online/free-courses/patient-centred-care (accessed 26 August 2022).

Hyde, E. and Hardy, M. (2020). Chapter 6 Patient centred care and considerations. In: *General Radiography: Principles and Practice* (ed. C. Hayre and W. Cox). London: CRC Press. https://www.routledge.com/General-Radiography-Principles-and-Practices/Hayre-Cox/p/book/9780367149871.

Hyde, E. and Hardy, M. (2021a). Delivering patient centred care (Part 1): Perceptions of service users and service deliverers. *Radiography* 27 (1): 8–13. https://doi.org/10.1016/j.radi.2020.04.015.

Hyde, E. and Hardy, M. (2021b). Delivering patient centred care (Part 2): A qualitative study of the perceptions of service users and deliverers. *Radiography* 27 (2): 322–331. https://doi.org/10.1016/j.radi.2020.09.008.

Hyde, E. and Hardy, M. (2021c). Delivering patient centred care (Part 3): Perceptions of student radiographers and radiography academics. *Radiography* 27 (3): 803–810. https://doi.org/10.1016/j.radi.2020.12.013.

Hyde, E. and Hardy, M. (2021d). Delivering informed measures of patient centred care in medical imaging: what is the international perspective? *Journal of Medical Imaging and Radiation Sciences*. Article in Press. https://doi.org/10.1016/j.jmir.2021.05.014.

Maslow, A.H. (1943). A theory of human motivation. *Psychological Review* 50 (4): 370–396.

Strudwick, R. and Hendry, J. (2021). Values-based practice. *Imaging & Therapy Pract* 11–15. ice.

Strudwick, R., Mackay, S., and Hicks, S. (2011). Is diagnostic radiography a caring profession? *Synergy* 4–7.

Strudwick, R., Newton-Hughes, A., Gibson, S. et al. (2018). Values-based practice (VBP) training for radiographers. https://www.sor.org/learning/document-library?page=1.

Taylor, A. and Hodgson, D. (2020). The behavioural display of compassion in radiation therapy: purpose, meaning and interpretation. *Journal of Medical Imaging and Radiation Sciences* 51 (2020): S59–S71. https://doi.org/10.1016/j.jmir.2020.08.003.

CHAPTER 15

Reflection on the Books and Skills Learned

Ruth M. Strudwick

Throughout this book we have explored some of the complex interpersonal skills required of radiotherapy practitioners and medical imaging professionals that enable the provision of high-quality person-centred care in radiography. This is based on the research, experiences, expertise, and interests of all the authors, and is targeted at all staff working within diagnostic and therapeutic radiography, whether in clinical departments or educational institutions. This includes radiographers, assistant practitioners, support workers, and administrative staff.

We hope that you have found it useful for your own practice to both teach others and to reflect on your own practice and develop your person-centred care skills.

We hope that you have been enabled to self-reflect, utilise the personal and professional development tools, and you feel more prepared to meet patients' expectations in clinical practice.

We hope that the activities, which are all based on evidence from our research, encourage you to reflect and discover how to apply what you have learned from this book to your own specific role. The scenarios demonstrate the impact of professional practitioners' behaviours and actions on patients'

Person-centred Care in Radiography: Skills for Providing Effective Patient Care, First Edition.
Ruth M. Strudwick, Jane M. Harvey-Lloyd, Jill Bleiker, Jane Gooch, Amy Hancock,
Emma Hyde, and Ann Newton-Hughes.
© 2024 John Wiley & Sons Ltd. Published 2024 by John Wiley & Sons Ltd.

perceptions of the care they have received and should allow you to make your own appraisal of what is meant by the terms 'person-centred' and 'values-based' practice – in practice!

We hope that in reading this book you feel better equipped to provide person-centred care for your patients, service users and their carers.

APPENDIX A

Organisational Measures of Patient Centred Care in Imaging Departments

Element	Considerations to be made:	Score 1 for each Yes, 0 for No
Accessing the Imaging Department	1. Are patients offered a choice of paper or electronic versions of their appointment letters?	Maximum score: 9
	2. Are appointment letters accompanied by relevant, understandable patient information about the examination?	
	3. Do the appointment letters provide any advice about what to wear, with the aim that patients do not need to change before their examination if they are appropriately attired?	
	4. Are appointment letters accompanied by maps showing the location of the Imaging department within the hospital?	

(Continued)

Person-centred Care in Radiography: Skills for Providing Effective Patient Care, First Edition.
Ruth M. Strudwick, Jane M. Harvey-Lloyd, Jill Bleiker, Jane Gooch, Amy Hancock,
Emma Hyde, and Ann Newton-Hughes.
© 2024 John Wiley & Sons Ltd. Published 2024 by John Wiley & Sons Ltd.

Element	Considerations to be made:	Score 1 for each Yes, 0 for No
	5. Are alternative versions of appointment letters and patient information available, such as different font sizes, Braille, or an alternative language?	
	6. Is there signage indicating the location of the imaging department from the hospital entrance/s, and main departments, such as Out Patient Clinic?	
	7. Is the signage clear and understandable to patients and/or carers?	
	8. Are greeters, volunteers, etc. on hand to offer directions, if required?	
	9. Is there an internal patient transport system which patients can use, if required?	
Waiting Areas	1. In the imaging department waiting areas, are there a range of seating styles and heights available to suit individual patient preferences/needs?	Maximum score: 9
	2. Are sub waiting areas available to accommodate individual patient needs, e.g. children's areas, in-patient areas, out-patient areas, quiet areas.	
	3. Are members of imaging department team visible and open to requests for help or information from patients and/or carers?	
	4. Are current waiting times or any delays in appointment times clearly communicated to patients and/or carers?	

Element	Considerations to be made:	Score 1 for each Yes, 0 for No
	5. Is there provision of water in waiting areas?	
	6. Is there a TV, with subtitles, in use in main waiting areas?	
	7. Is patient information provided on noticeboards, via posters or via leaflets in the waiting areas?	
	8. Is information provided on service improvement work based on patient feedback? *(Sometimes referred to as You Said It, We Did It)*	
	9. Are waiting areas organized to ensure health and safety of patients, staff and visitors, for example, are social distancing measures are in place, is PPE available, is hand sanitizer available, etc.?	
Professional interaction	1. Are all members of imaging department team welcoming and friendly?	Maximum score: 6
	2. Is 'Hello my name is . . .' used by all members of the Imaging department team?	
	3. Is patient confidentiality respected and maintained at the imaging department reception desk?	
	4. Do imaging department staff use appropriate language and/or terminology when talking to patients and/or carers?	
	5. Do imaging department staff encourage and answer questions from patients and/or carers appropriately?	

(Continued)

Element	Considerations to be made:	Score 1 for each Yes, 0 for No
	6. Is due care and attention paid to infection prevention and control measures?	
Availability and Style of Hospital Clothing	1. Is consideration given to whether patients need to change for their examination or not? 2. If patients need to change, are different sizes and/or styles of hospital gowns, dressing gowns, or alternatives to hospital gowns such as theatre scrubs or tracksuits available, to suit individual patient's needs? 3. If patients need to change, is assistance offered by a member of the imaging department team? 4. Do imaging department staff ensure that patients are suitably covered, and that their dignity is maintained?	Maximum score: 4
Availability and Style of Changing Rooms	1. Are changing rooms able to be secured, so that patients are not inadvertently exposed whilst changing? For example, do all changing room doors have locks? 2. Can patients enter the examination rooms directly from the changing rooms, to maintain their privacy and dignity? 3. Do waiting areas and changing areas have clean, modern décor? 4. Do waiting areas and changing areas have pictures or photographs of local beauty spots or landmarks?	Maximum score: 4

Element	Considerations to be made:	Score 1 for each Yes, 0 for No
Obtaining Results and Aftercare	1. At the end of the examination, is it clearly explained to the patient and/or carer what happens next?	Maximum score: 4
	2. Is appropriate advice provided to patients and/or carers about any aftercare required post examination, such as special dietary needs?	
	3. Is aftercare advice available in different formats, such as written, audio, Braille, in an alternative language, if required?	
	4. Are the results of imaging examinations available in a timely fashion? *(This item will need triangulating with departmental audits of reporting turnaround times)*	
Total score out of 36		**/36**

Score	Rating
30–36	Outstanding – patient-centred approaches are evident throughout the department. Only minor omissions.
21–29	Good – some good examples of patient-centred approaches, but some areas where improvements could be made.
15–20	Requires improvement – limited examples of patient-centred approaches, significant areas where improvements could be made.
Below 15	Inadequate – urgent action is needed to create a more patient-centred environment.

Pause and Check Audit Tool for Measuring Patient-Centred Care in Diagnostic Radiography (for use in Projection Radiography, Including Mammography)

Pre Examination Checklist		
Element	**Considerations to be made**	**Score 1 for each Yes, 0 for No**
Patient	1. Have you used 'Hello my name is ...' to introduce yourself to the patient and/or carer, and explained your role? 2. Have you asked the patient and/or carer how they wish to be addressed?	Maximum score: 7

Person-centred Care in Radiography: Skills for Providing Effective Patient Care, First Edition.
Ruth M. Strudwick, Jane M. Harvey-Lloyd, Jill Bleiker, Jane Gooch, Amy Hancock,
Emma Hyde, and Ann Newton-Hughes.
© 2024 John Wiley & Sons Ltd. Published 2024 by John Wiley & Sons Ltd.

Pre Examination Checklist		
Element	**Considerations to be made:**	**Score 1 for each Yes, 0 for No**
	3. Have you considered whether any adaptation of your communication style is required, e.g. visual cues, use of an interpreter, use of sign language, etc.?	
	4. Have you ensured that the patient and/or carer understands what is going to happen during the examination?	
	5. Have you provided an opportunity for the patient and/or carer to ask questions about the examination?	
	6. Have you gained informed consent before starting the examination?	
	7. Have you ensured that any instructions which need to be followed during the examination are audible to the patient, and considered whether any adaptation is required?	
Attire	1. Have you assessed whether the patient needs to change for their examination?	Maximum score: 2
	2. If the patient needs to change, have you offered assistance?	
	3. If the patient needs to change, have you considered appropriate gown sizes, the availability of dressing gowns, or the use of theatre scrubs to ensure the patient's privacy and dignity is maintained?	
User needs and wellbeing	1. Have you considered whether the patient has any specific needs which they may need support with during the examination?	Maximum score: 7

(Continued)

Pre Examination Checklist		
Element	**Considerations to be made:**	**Score 1 for each Yes, 0 for No**
	2. Has the patient been offered options to help support them during the examination, such as the presence of their carer? (Health and Safety permitting)	
Safety and Security	1. Have you considered how the patient can be supported to maintain the position needed for the examination safely, e.g. pillows, cushions, or pads?	Maximum score: 3
	2. Have you ensured the patient's belongings will be kept safe and secure for the duration of the examination?	
	3. Have infection prevention and control measures been considered?	
Environment	1. Have you asked the patient if they would like the lighting levels to be adjusted?	Maximum score: 2
	2. Have blankets or other ways to maintain warmth been offered?	
TOTAL out of 17		/17

During Examination Checklist		
Element	**Considerations to be made**	**Score 1 for each Yes, 0 for No**
Patient	1. Have you maintained communication with the patient during the examination, and established rapport with them? 2. Have you ensured that the patient and/or carer understand what is happening during the examination? 3. Have you provided continued opportunities for the patient and/or carer to ask questions about the examination?	Maximum score: 3
Attire	1. Have you ensured that the patient is appropriately covered by the clothing they are wearing for the examination at all times?	Maximum score: 1
User needs and wellbeing	1. Have you considered any specific needs the patient may have during the examination? 2. Have you provided the patient with options to help support them during the examination, such as the presence of their carer?	Maximum score: 2
Safety and Security	1. Have you ensured the patient is supported to maintain the position needed for the examination safely, using pillows, pads, sandbags, etc.? 2. Are the patient's belongings safe and secure for the duration of the examination?	Maximum score: 3

(Continued)

During Examination Checklist		
Element	**Considerations to be made**	**Score 1 for each Yes, 0 for No**
	3. Have you followed appropriate infection prevention and control measures?	
Environment	1. Have you checked the lighting levels are suitable for the patient?	Maximum score: 2
	2. Have you offered the patient blankets or other ways to maintain warmth?	
TOTAL out of 11		/11

Post Examination Checklist		
Element	**Considerations to be made**	**Score 1 for each Yes, 0 for No**
Patient	1. Have you allowed the patient time to sit up, restore their balance, etc. at the end of the examination?	Maximum score: 4
	2. Have you explained that the images are technically acceptable, but that a formal report needs to be written which will inform their results?	
	3. Have you ensured that the patient and/or carer understands how to get the results of the examination, and what will happen next?	
	4. Have you provided an opportunity for the patient and/or carer to ask questions?	

Post Examination Checklist		
Element	**Considerations to be made**	**Score 1 for each Yes, 0 for No**
Attire	1. Have you asked the patient if they need any assistance to change back into their own clothes?	Maximum score: 1
User needs and wellbeing	1. Have you asked whether the patient and/or carer need any assistance such as providing a wheelchair, calling for a porter, or notifying the ambulance service the patient is ready?	Maximum score: 3
	2. Have you checked whether the patient has any specific needs which they require support with, before leaving the department?	
	3. Have you considered signposting the patient and/or carer to any sources of additional support, e.g. Macmillan, Alzheimer's Society, etc.?	
Safety and Security	1. Have you provided information to the patient and/or carer about potential side effects due to the examination or aftercare advice?	Maximum score: 3
	2. Have you asked if the patient and/or carer has any questions about potential side effects or the aftercare advice?	
	3. Have you considered any safety aspects which may need to be highlighted to the patient and/or carer? For example, infection prevention and control measures.	

(Continued)

Post Examination Checklist		
Element	**Considerations to be made**	**Score 1 for each Yes, 0 for No**
Environment	1. Have you checked that the patient and/or carer knows the way out of the department? 2. Have you signposted the patient and/or carer to ways that they can provide feedback on their experience about the examination?	Maximum score: 2
TOTAL out of 13		/13
OVERALL TOTAL		/41

Score	Rating
38–41	Outstanding – patient centered approaches are evident throughout the examination. Only minor omissions.
30–37	Good – some good examples of patient centered approaches, but some areas of clinical practice where improvements could be made.
20–29	Requires improvement – some examples of patient centered approaches, significant areas of clinical practice where improvements could be made.
Below 20	Inadequate – urgent action is needed to embed patient centered approaches into clinical practice.

Index

Person-centred Care in Radiography: Skills for Providing Effective Patient Care, First Edition.
Ruth M. Strudwick, Jane M. Harvey-Lloyd, Jill Bleiker, Jane Gooch, Amy Hancock,
Emma Hyde, and Ann Newton-Hughes.
© 2024 John Wiley & Sons Ltd. Published 2024 by John Wiley & Sons Ltd.

Printed and bound by CPI Group (UK) Ltd, Croydon, CR0 4YY

24/09/2024

14562302-0001